The
Roy Adaptation
Model in Action

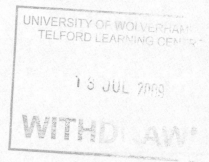

NURSING MODELS IN ACTION

The Roy Adaptation Model in Action

JUSTUS AKINSANYA
BSc, PhD, RN, ONC, BTA(Cert), RNT, FRCN, FWACN, FRSH
Pro Vice Chancellor and Dean
Anglia Polytechnic University

GREG COX
RN, RNT, DipN(Lond), RCNT(CertEd)
Lecturer in Nursing
Anglia Polytechnic University

CAROL CROUCH
BA, RN, RCNT, RNT(CertEd)
Lecturer in Nursing
Anglia Polytechnic University

and

LUCY FLETCHER
RN, DipN(Lond), RNT(CertEd(FE))
Lecturer in Nursing
University of Hertfordshire

Series Editor
BOB PRICE

M

MACMILLAN

First published 1994 by
THE MACMILLAN PRESS LTD
Houndmills, Basingstoke, Hampshire RG21 2XS
and London
Companies and representatives
throughout the world

ISBN 0-333-57414-1

A catalogue record for this book is available
from the British Library

Printed in Great Britain by Mackays of Chatham PLC, Chatham, Kent

CONTENTS

v

It is a privilege to introduce this volume on the Roy Adaptation Model in the series Nursing Models in Action. To link conceptual developments with nursing practice provides such theorising with a reason for being. We think about nursing and what it means only to provide effective practice.

There is no doubt that in this endeavour, the nurse is reflective, however, as the authors have so clearly noted, it is the model that provides the guidelines for reflection. This reminds me of an incident that occurred a few years ago when I was a participant at a nursing theory conference at the Royal College of Nursing in London. As might be expected at any such conference, there were sceptics among the audience. After hours of presentations and discussions, a ray of light broke through the murkiness.

One participant shared a profound insight, 'Oh, I get it; when we were told to use the nursing process, we should have had nursing models first, to know what we are processing'. Yes, truly the nursing process is a hollow skill. It assumes that the nurse processes with the patient the assessment, planning, implementation and evaluation that is individualised nursing.

The model of nursing provides an answer to the questions, what is nursing about and therefore, what is the nurse about when doing nursing? This crucial link between the concepts of the model and how the nurse manages each patient situation is apparent throughout the chapters of this book.

The authors have demonstrated this link of models to nursing practice in repeated real clinical situations. This provides a real service for believers and sceptics alike.

A second fundamental issue to which the authors contribute some clarity is the question of the use of theories and models in curriculum development. The rationale for the place of models in nursing education is the same as that for their use in practice.

To teach about nursing, one knowingly or unknowingly takes a stance on one's beliefs and concepts of nursing. Models provide both the organising framework and direction for the detail that is taught in the classroom, the laboratory and the practice branches. A word of encouragement is warranted here. Countless faculties have debated the ponderous issues of major change. To undertake this arduous task takes commitment to both the heritage of nursing and to the principles one wants to operationalise. This is not a project for the faint-hearted. Yet no matter how difficult the task, your colleagues in similar endeavours can assure you that the outcome is exceedingly rewarding. The professional growth of nursing among new nurses and those working with them soon becomes obvious. Nursing does not essentially change, but rather becomes manifest and explicable.

Finally, the openness and stance of critique that the authors uphold are to be commended. The authors' concern that we maintain a critical stance in the use and study of nursing models is pivotal. Models are useful in the extent to which they guide effective nursing practice and raise further questions to be solved in practice. A closed and stylised system is not immediately receptive to new ideas because there is a tendency to reinterpret any observations to make them conform to the system [Fleck, L. (1979) *Genesis and Development of a Scientific Fact*, Chicago, Illinois: University of Chicago]. However, nursing knowledge develops as does all knowledge. We allow room for error because discovery is inextricably interwoven with being able to recognise a new relation. To recognise this new relation, many another relation must be denied or overlooked. We can say that the practice situation can be described in a given way by the model. But the model itself is developing and this growth may call for additional identification of new relations.

A good example that the authors note is the understanding of the regular and cognator mechanisms. These theoretical concepts are used to describe the process central to human adaptation. Using careful observations in practice, and skilful research design, the basic dynamics of this adaptive process can come to light. Nurses can identify some of the commonalities in cognator/regulator activity in patients. Differences in such activity from person to person can be studied. A much fuller science of the person awaits such detailed work.

We are pleased to have colleagues on both sides of the Atlantic working on the professional expression of nursing in education, practice and research. We hope that nursing models may provide the fullest of contribution to this effort.

Boston, Massachusetts, USA   SISTER CALLISTA ROY
                                                RN, PhD, FAAN

Whether we are referring to changes in society, professional practice, or the technological and economic challenges facing nurses and patients alike, we are all familiar with the need for 'adaptation' – at least in a passing way. Adaptation, coping, developing, thriving and growing are the parlance of everyday conversations, the concerns of parents and spouses, and the goals of nursing. Nevertheless, there is immeasurable benefit in organising such ideas, and the Roy model of adaptation and nursing practice achieves this. Working with her experiences of cancer patients, and a philosophy of human nature that emphasises endeavour and ability to change, Roy developed a model that has achieved widespread acceptance both within her native United States of America, and across the nursing world.

While Roy's adaptation model has been widely welcomed by nurses, there remains a need to understand it as a whole, and in contexts beyond a single culture of clinical circumstance. If the model is to have relevance to the profession it must offer wisdom beyond rehabilitation settings, and to nurses at all levels of practice. Achieving this dual aim, actioning the model, while reserving the right to pass critical evaluation, have been the purposes of this text. In common with its series companions, it sets out to provide a clear and pragmatic guide to nursing theory, and the extent to which it can inform clinical decisions, care negotiation and professional practice in general.

Recently, the vogue for developing 'reflective practice' has tended to overshadow some aspects of such theory. Intuitive expertise, reflection in action, during the process of care planning and delivering, has become a subject for nursing debate. It can be argued that there is less need for a nursing model. If expert care is largely intuitive, circumstantial and trait related, perhaps nursing models cease to offer guidance to practice? On the other hand however, before experts can emerge, it is usually accepted that they need to formulate ways of thinking about clinical problems. There is a need for models to assist learners as they evolve practice that blends theory and experience, in order to judge when and where to break with convention and offer a different approach.

Whether we believe the nurse is largely intuitive or rational and analytic in her approach to care, Roy's model affords one set of guidance notes to inspire and prompt flexible attitudes to practice. Offering as it does encouragement to deeper assessment (stimuli and behaviour), a closer professional relationship, and a greater understanding of physiology (regulator functions) and psychology (cognator functions), it remains a thoroughly modern and relevant model with which to practise. However much we may demur at terminology, or debate nursing roles, few would argue about the central place of adaptation during illness. For this reason, if no other, Roy's model retains a central and well-founded place within the nursing curriculum.

Professor Akinsanya, Greg Cox, Carol Crouch and Lucy Fletcher offer a wide-ranging review of the model and apply it to both circumstances of health and illness. They have not been afraid to explore its potential at each stage of the problem-solving process, nor to test its structure and clarity with patients who offer multiple problems. There is a fresh excitement evident as they apply the model, and ample opportunity to measure the link of theory to practice, stretching across the Atlantic, and from hospital to home. Each of the care studies authenticates Roy's theory in action, and retains some expression of the individual practitioner's way of giving care.

It is as if there is a conceptual tool kit, a resource to be drawn upon. Nevertheless, like all reflective practitioners, these nurses have retained the right to make local decisions, based upon experience as well as model guidance. I hope that as you read through the care studies it will become as apparent to you as it was to me – using a model effectively and sensitively is what good nursing is all about. There is no need to turn models, concepts or theories into dogma – whether that be adaptation, reflection or caring.

BOB PRICE
SRN, BA, MSc, CertEd(FE), ARRC
Series Editor

ACKNOWLEDGEMENTS

The preparation of this book began during the most challenging period in British nursing education. The implementation of the Project 2000 proposals depended on links being established between Schools of Nursing and higher education. One of the authors, Justus Akinsanya, delivered a professorial inaugural lecture in 1988 in which he argued that nursing education should be fully integrated into higher education rather than remain outside it.

In October 1992, Anglia Polytechnic University duly brought together all schools of nursing and midwifery in mid, west and south Essex into an integrated Faculty of Health and Social Work. The authors had come together two years earlier to plan and develop ideas for this book.

First and foremost, we would like to thank Bob Price, the Series Editor, for his constructive, incisive and sensitive approach to the demands we made on him. He supported us enthusiastically and was always willing to help sort out otherwise seemingly intractable problems during the writing of this book. Kerry Lawrence, of Macmillan Press, regularly reminded us of our deadlines and her patience is warmly acknowledged.

We are grateful to Sister Callista Roy, the originator of the model, for writing the Foreword to the book. The conceptual clarity of her theoretical thinking challenged us to seek to put the model into action. In doing so, we have gained much from colleagues in the Faculty and within clinical areas. We owe a debt of gratitude to the patients and clients whose care needs shaped our thinking in applying the model as described in the book.

Brenda Marlow and Hiedi Yetton helped in manuscript preparation in a number of ways for which we are grateful. Finally, we would like to pay particular tribute and express our gratitude to our families for their support and patience during the long period of preparing the manuscript for publication.

JUSTUS AKINSANYA
GREG COX
CAROL CROUCH
LUCY FLETCHER

CHAPTER ONE

General introduction
Justus Akinsanya

What is a nursing theory? A definition of nursing theory given by Stevens (1984) notes that it is an 'attempt to describe or explain the phenomenon called nursing.' This definition, though helpful, is nevertheless inadequate, for nursing is not strictly a phenomenon but rather a widely recognised activity. It is therefore important for those coming to the study of nursing theories for the first time, to add that a nursing theory not only describes and explains what nurses do but, as Jacox (1974) points out, also gives guidance for action needed to meet nursing goals. Table 1.1 summarises the definitions used by theorists.

A nursing theory, therefore, has three important components which are concerned with:

- description of nursing goals in the light of identified individual needs for care;
- explanation of planned nursing intervention based on appropriate knowledge;
- prescription of nursing action.

One emerging theme in any consideration of theories of nursing is that they should be unique to nursing if they are to be called nursing theories. Indeed, Stevens (1984) argues that: 'It is important that any given nursing theory – directly or by implication – differentiates nursing from other disciplines and activities.' This means that nursing theory should identify those characteristics which are separate from medicine or social work, for example, or from non-professional activities such as mothering or nurturing. Although this uniqueness is important, it must be appreciated that nursing borrows

Table 1.1 *Definitions used in theory development*

Term	Definition
Concept	An abstraction representing a classification usually of a single description/definition of some entity, e.g. homeostasis. It clarifies some aspects of a body of knowledge and is used as a building block for conceptual ideas.
Proposition	This is a single statement used to relate two or more concepts. It defines the relationship between concepts and gives them a clear focus for understanding their application. For example, the two concepts of homeostasis and adaptation can be related by a proposition which describes how they may affect each other in real life. The relationship so described may be untested but it represents the beginning of a testable statement.
Theory	This is a group or set of propositions which are interrelated in some systematic way. A theory provides a basis for organising knowledge and using it to guide the way we deal with life events on the basis of its underlying assumptions.
Hypothesis	This is a relationship proposition or statement which can be empirically tested. It defines a specific relationship between the stated concepts which can then be tested using the scientific method. It is important in the testing of theories. For example, Hayward's (1975) study tested the hypothesis that pre-operative information and the preception of post-operative pain are related. On the basis of this hypothesis, it was predicted that patients given information about their operation pre-operatively will experience less pain following surgery and thus require less analgesic.
Conceptual model	This is a unified, concrete representation of a concept. It provides a structured and organised conceptual relationship that is possible in a 'conceptual framework' (see below). Model building is an important method of investing an idea with the demands of reality.
Conceptual framework	The interrelationships between concepts, described loosely, in order to provide a structure to guide the development of testable hypotheses.
Theoretical framework	A conceptual model containing both structure and detail. It brings together the structure and function of a theory by explaining its constituent elements.

knowledge from many other disciplines such as the life and behavioural sciences. For this reason, nursing science is an applied science, i.e. a blend of knowledge from other sciences. This borrowing of knowledge from other sciences does not mean that nursing theory cannot be unique since it can be argued that the very nature of its mix of the sciences which underpin its art constitutes such a uniqueness. It should also be noted that nursing theory is unique not just in the blend of its knowledge base, but also in the use and application of that knowledge. It is now clear that although nursing shares a focus with medicine, psychology and social work (in that they all study man and health), each discipline has a different frame of reference and applies its knowledge in a unique way. For instance, medicine emphasises health promotion through prevention and cure of disease processes. Nursing also has a preventive component but its restoration of health is achieved through caring for the individual.

DEVELOPMENT OF THEORIES OF NURSING

The background to the development of nursing theories has been explored by a number of writers. Newton (1991) relates the development to the emerging role of women in Western society while Cavanagh (1991) points to the influence of nursing as an academic discipline in the USA. There are two ways in which the development of nursing theories may be considered – the *deductive approach* and the *inductive approach*.

Deductive approach

As noted earlier, theoretical ideas can be borrowed from other disciplines and applied to nursing. For example, if a nursing theory is to be applied to the prevention and healing of pressure sores, it is important to examine the causes and processes of tissue breakdown and the pathological events leading to the regeneration of tissue. The knowledge for this approach is derived from the biological theory of *homeostasis*, which can be used to identify those types of nursing where intervention is appropriate and those where it is not.

Thus by applying the knowledge from pathology to a nursing situation, the nurse is helping in the development of a nursing theory by the deductive method. The theory which underpins the understanding of pressure necrosis as a nursing problem is validated empirically, i.e. by carrying out a study to test the theory. The development of Norton's scale for judging the vulnerability of individuals to pressure sores (Norton *et al.*, 1975) derives from this application of the concept of homeostasis from physiology.

Inductive approach

A nursing theory can also be developed through a close examination of an area of nursing practice, identifying the components and relationships, and testing and validating the efficacy of that practice by research. For example, a nurse might notice that despite regular timing some of her patients are still developing pressure sores. On close examination she identifies that other factors are present, such as weight loss, poor nutritional status, incontinence or oedema. She then undertakes a descriptive study on all immobile patients, documenting the characteristics of those patients who develop sores and those who do not. She identifies the risk factors, plans appropriate nursing care and then evaluates whether her change in nursing intervention has any effect on the number of pressure sores that her patients develop.

These two examples based on deductive and inductive approaches to theory development demonstrate a similar pattern in that they contain the four levels of theory development discussed by Dickoff *et al.* (1968). The authors suggest that, in any attempt to develop a theory, the following are the essential levels of a theory-building exercise:

1. isolation of factors by naming and putting them into different categories;
2. recognition of relationships between factors;
3. decision on situations in which recognised relationships occur – thus future events may be predicted, promoted or inhibited;
4. prescription of outcomes based on a situation-producing theory in which goals are set and activities are planned and carried out in order to meet the goals.

The authors suggest that 'nursing theory, if it is to have an impact on practice, must be theory at the most sophisticated level, namely a situation-producing theory.'

THEORY, THEORETICAL FRAMEWORKS AND CONCEPTUAL MODELS

It has become increasingly clear in recent years that most nurses are unclear about the meanings of different terms used in discuss-

4

ing theories of nursing. Griffith-Kenny and Christensen (1987) note that terms such as theory, theoretical framework and conceptual models 'are frequently used indiscriminately and interchangeably in nursing and in other disciplines. These terms have been defined differently by various writers, and this has led to a great deal of confusion.'

In order to clear up this apparent confusion, the authors describe a model as a group of concepts, ideas or themes that are interrelated, but in which the relationships are not clearly defined. Theoretical frameworks, on the other hand, are generally less broader than models but are more so than in a theory.

Models are essential guides to theory development while conceptual frameworks provide the theorist with specified concepts as focal points. Because these ideas are fundamental prerequisites for theory development, it is not surprising that much time is devoted to their analysis (Akinsanya, 1984; 1989). Thus Riehl and Roy (1980) examined the relationship between models and theory and noted that 'the term model is broader than the term theory when applied to nursing.' In all scientific undertakings, the construction of a model is a useful exercise. It gives a broad image of the entire field under consideration. This is true of nursing in which models are constructed in order to relate different parts of the discipline and thus enable the theorist to describe, explain and indeed predict the effects of their application to the practice of nursing.

ROY AND THE ELEMENTS OF NURSING MODELS

Roy (1976) suggests that all nursing models have common, shared elements. However, the interpretation of these elements differs between each model. The elements she identified are:

1. *The recipient of nursing care.*   Each model has its own view of man as the recipient of care.
2. *The goal of nursing.*   Within each model, the purpose or goal of nursing reflects the view of man as a goal-seeking being.
3. *Nursing activity.*   The nursing action described in each model reflects the model's particular view of man and the nursing goals. In an attempt to highlight commonalities rather than differences, an important scientific exercise, Aggleton and Chalmers (1984) have listed the features common to all nursing models and they state that such a list provides a framework by which different models and their emphases can be compared. When reading about Roy's Adaptation Model in subsequent chapters, the reader should

try to identify the common elements as described above and their application in the clinical setting.

PURPOSE OF NURSING THEORIES AND MODELS

Before describing and examining Roy's Adaptation Model, it is important for the reader to reflect on the controversy surrounding the use of theories in nursing. A recurring question from those who require evidence for their usefulness is whether nursing theories and models serve any practical purpose. In order to answer this question, it is necessary to look at the alternative to using them. In recent years, a number of authors have argued that the use of medically oriented perspective has limited the opportunity for nursing to develop its own theoretical foundation. Indeed, Adam (1983) has suggested that consciously or not, nursing practice, education and research have been guided by the same conceptual reference as has medicine. Such a frame of reference has been termed the 'medical model' and it is still being used widely.

In this model the patient is depicted as a diseased person who exhibits signs and symptoms. The nurse who uses such a model is seen as one who records signs and symptoms, reports them to the medical staff and carries out their orders for treatment as shown in Figure 1.1 (Akinsanya and Hayward, 1980; Chapman, 1985). Such a model has also been used in education where nurses learn about 'the nursing care of patients with myocardial infarctions' or 'the

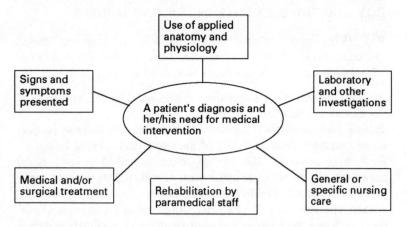

Figure 1.1 *Features of the Medical Model. In this model, nursing care is one of the factors taken into account by the medical practitioner*

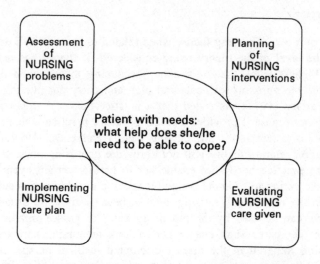

Figure 1.2 *Features of the Nursing Model. Although often described as the 'nursing process', it should be noted that assessing, planning, implementing and evaluating are logical steps employed in the decision-making process in all aspects of life*

nursing care of patients after an appendicectomy'. This should be compared with the nursing model in which patients' problems are assessed, care is planned and implemented, and finally evaluated for effectiveness. (Figure 1.2).

Adam (1983) argued that if nurses are to use the medical rather than the nursing model, the very professional foundation for autonomous practice would be called into question. She argues that such an approach would mean that nurses should ' . . . cease referring to their profession as an autonomous one . . . and . . . stop talking about a body of nursing knowledge and about advancing nursing science.' Others such as Cornellius (1977) see the issue in terms of accountability for nursing action while Lynaugh and Bates (1973) suggested that the language of medicine and nursing are in any event different, hence their perspectives should not be confused.

Thus the purpose of nursing theories and models is to give professional expression to three main areas of nursing – its education, practice and research.

Practice

The purpose of nursing theory when related to practice will depend on the level of the theory being considered. If theory has reached the highest level, that of situation-producing theory, then it will enable the nurse to set goals and plan and carry out nursing care. McFarlane (1977) has stated that a practice theory is important to nursing because it provides a prescription for practice which in her view 'is where, after all, nursing begins and ends.' However, a situation-relating theory will not allow the practising nurse to prescribe practice but rather enable her to predict certain events and to take action to promote or inhibit specific events from occurring.

On the other hand, nursing models, because they are broader in scope, can be used by the practising nurse to guide, organise and direct her care. They enable her to look at nursing care from a nursing rather than the disease-orientated medical perspective. It would be reasonable to suggest, therefore, that nurses require such a framework to guide, organise and direct them in the assessment, identification of nursing problems, and the planning and evaluation of the care they give to their patients. In other words, a nursing model, by virtue of its wider application, provides a unifying theme or framework for the organisation of nursing knowledge and its application to practice.

The importance of application cannot be over-emphasised and Clark (1982) suggests that using models and theories in nursing 'has practical value for the ordinary clinical nurse, as a tool which she can use to help her look critically at her own practice to improve the effectiveness of the care she gives.' For Clark, the main purpose of theory development in nursing is the 'improvement of the service to patients.'

Education

There are two areas in nursing education where nursing models and theories can be of use. Firstly, models and theories are useful to the nursing student in relation to a professional orientation to the discipline itself. Thus nursing theory and models are aids to increase the understanding of what nursing is and of what nurses do. There is a body of evidence from educational research to support the view that theories and models can assist the clarity of abstract ideas and thus assist in the learning process. Certainly, they give a framework within which knowledge can be organised and stored in mind for use. This simplifies retrieval of information. It could therefore be argued that the curriculum should include more than one model so that they can be compared with each other. Such a comparison could help the student to examine nursing concepts more critically.

Nevertheless, the use of theories and models in nursing education is generally rudimentary. It would seem appropriate that learners be introduced to a good model during their training in order to provide them with a foundation for thinking theoretically about nursing and the subsequent application of theory to practice. It could also be argued that such an early introduction to rigour and a critical approach to theory development and application would assist learners in differentiating between what is good and what is bad practice in nursing.

Secondly, nursing models and theories are useful to the nurse teacher for they can provide a framework for curriculum development. In recent years, they have been used as pointers to relevant areas to be included in the curriculum and as links or themes which run through specific courses. The Roper *et al.* (1990) model for nursing has been introduced into a number of nursing curricula in the United Kingdom because it provides a guidance for teachers when preparing courses in basic nursing education. The application of the Roper *et al.*'s activities of living in the design of curricula is now widely used in the United Kingdom.

All these point to a deliberate desire to avoid using a medical model, and Weatherson (1979) has pointed out that 'the curriculum which focuses on disease will not encourage regard of the individual as a whole person.' Yet there are difficulties in this approach, for the nurse should be able to apply theory learned in the school to the practice situation. If the system used in practice is based on the medical model, then the introduction of a nursing model into the curriculum will increase the disenchantment that the student experiences when confronted with the discrepancies between theory and practice.

Research

Nursing research can be guided by models and theories of nursing. Two of the contributors to theory development in nursing, Riehl and Roy (1980), state that 'Throughout the total research process, from definition of the problem through confirmation or negation of the hypothesis, the nursing model provides guidance.' However,

9

it is important to stress that the choice of a model is crucial in that the nature of the problem being investigated would determine the type of model to be used in guiding its investigation. Moreover, the techniques and research tools to be employed and the setting in which research is conducted and data gathered (and their later analysis) will all depend on a theoretical framework or model upon which the research is to be based.

Although research depends on a foundation of a theoretical framework, Fawcett (1989) has argued that the use of nursing models may be limited because of the difficulty in testing them empirically. This difficulty may arise where concepts within a model are too abstract in nature so that real-life testing becomes difficult. The major problem appears to lie in the fact that nursing science is still young and, as Fawcett pointed out, it 'is essentially devoid of any substantive nursing themes that could be related to nursing research.'

NURSING THEORIES AND MODELS – IMPLICATIONS FOR PRACTICE, EDUCATION AND RESEARCH

For reasons of clarity, the previous section examined how nursing theories and models can influence practice, education and research. This approach was adopted in order to establish the purpose of nursing theories and models in that context. However, the relationship between these concepts is more complex since practice, education and research all exert an influence singly or collectively on the development and use of nursing theories and models. They also influence the way theorists see the conceptual interrelationships between these aspects of nursing. It is therefore important to be aware of these influences when considering the nature and purpose of theories of nursing.

SUMMARY

This introductory chapter has sought to explain the way in which theories and models differ, as well as to identify their common features. The theories and modes of nursing clearly have purpose in so far as they provide frameworks for the systematic development of a knowledge-based practice. It is interesting to note that all theoretical considerations in nursing over the past three decades have not produced one single, unifying and all-encompassing theory or model suited to all specialities. Indeed, the reader should be clear that none of the existing conceptions of nursing has received universal acceptance. Nor is it desirable that this should be so, because knowledge is cumulative and ever-changing and no scientific pursuit is static. For this reason, the search for a universal theory may not be necessary. Wright (1986) comments that 'The one theory, one model, one way approach is a narrow dogma we should avoid.'

What is true is that a number of concepts have been adopted by nurse theorists based on knowledge derived from other disciplines where their truth had been universally established and acknowledged. Thus concepts such as 'self-care' and 'adaptation' are useful in helping to identify areas of nursing concern. As McFarlane (1977) noted, the existence of many concepts within nursing theories may reflect a lack of consensus in the profession, but they may also reflect the complexity of the practice and its underlying fundamental assumptions. So, to the question as to which theories or which models nurses choose in their education, practice and research, Altschul (1979) gives the following advice:

'Let nurses use what models seem productive in their search for greater understanding of whatever it is they do.'

In the consideration of the nature and purpose of theories of nursing, this seems an eminently valuable advice to guide the practising nurse, educator or researcher. It also provides a justification for the indepth discussion of Roy's Adaptation Model in this book, and of the efforts to provide examples of its use in clinical practice.

REFERENCES

Adam, E. (1983) Frontiers of nursing in the 21st century: development of models and theories on the concept of nursing. *Journal of Advanced Nursing*, **8**(1), 41–45.

Aggleton, P. and Chalmers, H. (1984) Defining the terms. *Nursing Times*, 5 September, pp. 24–28.

Akinsanya, J. A. (1984) The uses of theories in nursing. *Nursing Times*, **80**(14), 59–60.

Akinsanya, J. A. (Ed.) (1989) *Theories and Models of Nursing* (Recent Advances in Nursing). Edinburgh: Churchill Livingstone.

Akinsanya, J. A. and Hayward, J. C. (1980) Biological sciences in nursing education: a bionursing approach. *Nursing Times*, **76**(10), 427–432.

Altschul, A. T. (1979) Commitment to nursing. *Journal of Advanced Nursing*, **4**(2), 123–135.

Cavanagh, S. J. (1991) *Orem's Model in Action*. London: Macmillan.

Chapman, C. (1985) *Theory of Nursing: Practical Application*. London: Harper & Row.

Clark, J. (1982) Development of models and theories on the concept of nursing. *Journal of Advanced Nursing*, 7(2), 129–134.

Cornellius, D. (1977) *Presidential Address at the ICN 16th Quadrennial Congress*, Tokyo, Japan.

Dickoff, J., James, P. and Wiedenbach, E. (1968) Theory in a practice discipline. *Nursing Research*, 17, 415–554.

Fawcett, J. (1989) *Analysis and Evaluation of Conceptual Models in Nursing*, 2nd edn. Philadelphia, Pennsylvania: F. A. Davis.

Griffith-Kenny, J. W. and Christensen, P. J. (1987) *Nursing Process: Application of Theories, Frameworks and Models*, 2nd edn. St Louis, Missouri: Mosby.

Hayward, J. C. (1975) *Information: A Prescription Against Pain*. London: Royal College of Nursing.

Jacox, A. (1974) Theory construction in nursing: an overview. *Nursing Research*, **23j**(1), 4–13.

Lynaugh, J. E. and Bates, B. (1973) The two languages of medicine and nursing. *American Journal of Nursing*, **73**, 66–69.

McFarlane, J. K. (1977) Developing a theory of nursing: the relation of theory to practice, education and research. *Journal of Advanced Nursing*, **2**(3), 261–270.

Newton, C. (1991) *The Roper–Logan–Tierney Model in Action*. London: Macmillan.

Norton, D., McLaren, R. and Exton-Smith, A. N. (1975) *An Investigation of Geriatric Nursing Problems in Hospital*. Edinburgh: Churchill Livingstone.

Riehl, J. P. and Roy, C. (1980) *Conceptual Models for Nursing Practice*, 2nd edn. Norwalk, Connecticut: Appleton-Century Croft.

Roper, N., Logan, W. and Tierney, A. (1990) *The Elements of Nursing, a Model for Nursing based on a Model of Living*, 3rd edn. Edinburgh: Churchill Livingstone.

Roy, C. (1976) *Introduction to Nursing: An Adaptation Model*. Englewood Cliffs, New Jersey: Prentice-Hall.

Stevens, B. J. (1984) *Nursing Theory: Analysis, Application and Evaluation*. Boston, Massachusetts: Little, Brown.

Weatherson, L. (1979) Theories of nursing: creating effective care. *Journal of Advanced Nursing*, **4**(4), 365–375.

Wright, S. (1986) *Building and Using a Model of Nursing*. London: Edward Arnold.

CHAPTER TWO

Introduction to Roy Adaptation Model
Justus Akinsanya

Adaptation is a biological concept and is the basis for the fundamental concept of homeostasis which is widely used in the study of biology. Adaptation relates to the way an individual responds to changes in the environment whereas homeostasis is concerned with the internal environment. It is important at the outset to be clear about the importance of adaptation and how, using this concept, Sister Callista Roy had developed her model which is designed, as with all conceptual models in nursing, to guide its practice.

The model was introduced by the author in 1970 following a period of intellectual development of ideas about nursing and how best to provide a conceptual framework for its practice. It was completed in 1984. The Adaptation Model uses an approach which focuses on the individuals who may be experiencing difficulties in coping with changes in their lives. The cornerstone of its contribution to the theoretical framework for nursing is its use of a problem-solving approach designed to assist and support people in achieving adaptive states consequent upon changes in their environments.

An important aspect of any theory is that assumptions have to be made in setting basic parameters for an understanding of its underlying concepts, principles and their later application to practical problems. In this case, the following underlying assumptions are attributed to the development of Roy's model:

- the individual is a bio-psycho-social being;
- individuals use innate and acquired mechanisms which are biological, psychological and social in origin;

- there is a constant interaction between the individual and the environment which calls for adaptive responses;
- health and illness occur in a continuum and the individual may experience both in the course of a life time;
- environmental changes call for individual adaptive responses;
- the individual's adaptive response is a function of the level of stimulus, and responses are dependent on the level of adaptation achieved;
- the response to a stimulus depends on its strength and the zone on which it falls in the body;
- there are four modes of adaptation which determine the individual's responses to stimuli, as shown in Figure 2.1.

Riehl and Roy (1980) describe two levels of assessment in applying the model in the planning of nursing care. The *first level of assessment* concerns the identification of the patient's adaptive behaviour which must be positive and effective in overcoming changes in the environment. On the other hand, the individual's adaptive behaviour may be maladjusted and ineffective, giving rise to individual experiences which are negative and problematic. This level of assessment is essential in determining individual needs as a basis for any planned nursing intervention.

The *second level of assessment* relates to the identification of the stimuli which influenced the development of particular adaptive behaviour in the individual. As with the first level of assessment, the individual may show positive adaptive behaviour or be maladaptive in response to the changes in the environment.

The nature of the stimulus may be defined in three ways:

1. *Focal* stimuli refer to those which are immediate in their impact and which require the individual to respond rapidly. A focal stimulus therefore confronts the individual with a requirement for immediate response in order to adjust to the changing environment.
2. *Contextual* stimuli are those which contribute to the overall response by the individual. These occur alongside the focal stimuli and may influence adaptive responses from the individual.
3. *Residual* stimuli are those others which are not validated by immediate experience of the individual but owe their contribution to the past experiences, beliefs or attitudes.

These stimuli are maintained by two sets of processes which determine their effectiveness in eliciting responses from the individual. The first of these is *stimuli regulator* which is largely autonomic and is therefore dependent on the functioning of the nervous and hormonal systems. The second, called a cognator, relates to the conscious process of thought and decision which the individual controls in response to internal and external changes. The process of homeostasis is internally maintained by both nervous and hormonal changes while adaptive responses to changes in the external environment require conscious decisions by the individual.

MODES IN ROY'S MODEL

The physiological mode is concerned with the structure and functions of the body. It relates the morphological differentiation of cells, tissues and organs to the systems they constitute and how the functions they sustain affect the adaptive behaviour of the individual. When changes occur internally, the body is stimulated to respond in order to adapt to the changes. The response to changes in the physiological mode is related to homeostasis and is affected by, among other responses, those concerned with:

- oxygen and circulation;
- fluid and electrolyte balance;
- nutrition;
- elimination;
- rest and activity;
- regulation of body functions (e.g. temperature).

In general, needs within the physiological mode of adaptation may have other consequences for the individual and lead to such responses as:

- hyperactivity;
- fatigue;
- malnutrition;
- vomiting;
- constipation;
- incontinence;
- dehydration;
- oedema;
- electrolyte imbalance;
- oxygen deficit/excess;
- shock;
- fever − hypothermia;
- sensory deprivation/overload;
- endocrine imbalance.

15

As with other theoretical innovations in nursing during the past three decades, the need for a link between theory and practice in nursing was recognised by nurses based in academic establishments who were interested in the development of a knowledge base for practice. Roy's Adaptation Model makes an important contribution to the development of theoretical ideas and their uses as a framework for nursing practice.

Roy's model is concerned with the problem of human adaptation. She suggested that the human organism consists of parts which depend for their existence and survival on an integrated functioning of the whole body. The parts which make up the whole, therefore, are linked together in a dynamic equilibrium such that any change to one part (or force applied to it) would lead to reaction which would ultimately affect the whole organism. The force could be biological, psychological or social. Hence the central concept of the model is that of man as a 'bio-psycho-social' being.

In order to understand the way in which the Model (and others in the series) affect practical issues in nursing, it is important to be clear about the terminology used by the theorists. This is summarised in Table 1.1 of Chapter 1.

The view that man is a bio-psycho-social being in constant interaction with his environment and adapting as appropriate is known as the concept of 'homeostasis' in the study of biological sciences. It could also be argued that there are psychological and social equilibria which are maintained in response to external and internal pressures on the human body. As shown in Figure 2.1, there are concepts and principles which relate to the ideas developed and applied by Roy in her Model. The application of the Model is illustrated in Figures 2.1 and 2.2.

CONCEPT OF MODES

Roy uses the concept of modes outlined above to describe four aspects of her model and to provide a link with the reality of practice. In any attempt to systematise the application of a concept, it is important for a clear link to be provided between conceptual thinking and the practical application of the concept. In this model, Roy suggests that the modes may be classified within two specific levels of assessment.

It should be remembered that, in using the Nursing Process or what Roper *et al.* (1990) describe as the Process of Nursing, assessment is the first point of the process in which the nurse attempts

16

Figure 2.1   *Illustrative summary of application of key concepts in Roy's Adaptation Model*

Mrs Sampson is a 66-year-old woman who was discharged home following the reduction of a fractured neck of her left femur. She lives alone in a flat and spends most of her time in bed because she feels a lot of pain when moving. When the district nurse called on her one morning, Mrs Sampson reported that she had not eaten 'for days'. She was weak and had lost some weight. She was constipated and in considerable pain.

Example of the use of Roy's Model in the planning of Mrs Sampson's care

Short-term objectives:

- Mrs Sampson will be pain free in 48–72 hours;
- she will show interest in eating and drinking again and will maintain adequate nutrition;
- she will be able to get around her flat confidently with the use of a walking stick after pain control is achieved;
- she will learn to adapt her limited independence when carrying out activities of living;
- she will alter her adaptation levels in the context of her new dependency;
- she will be aware of the social activities in her area for recreation and companionship.

First-stage assessment – physiological adaptive mode:

- Actual problems – pain, immobility, weakness, poor nutrition and constipation

Self-concept adaptive mode:

- Actual problems – powerless, anxiety and loss of confidence in body image

Role function adaptive mode:

- Actual Problems – failure to carry out role expected by hospital (due to injury) and herself (due to pain and her home condition)

---

to locate the nursing problems of the patient. Thus in classifying the modes within her model, Roy makes a number of assumptions as follows:

- the nature of adaptation as a biological means of survival;
- man is a bio-psycho-social being;
- man is an interactionist;
- man responds to changes in his environment;

17

Figure 2.2   *Modes of adaptation in Roy's Model: interdependency mode*

Example of application in practice:

• Actual problems – sense of rejection and loneliness

Nature of stimuli

Focal – stimuli immediately affecting Mrs Sampson, i.e. loss of independence but hospital expected her to cope alone at home.

Contextual – stimuli occurring alongside the focal which may influence adaptation to focal stimulus, e.g. her poor environment. The sick role was reinforced in the hospital.

Residual – stimuli remaining from the past which may affect her ability to adapt, e.g. beliefs, attitudes and experiences of similar painful stimuli.

• Actual problem – feeling of rejection and loneliness. Had been sent home when she believed and felt she was still ill and responding to the sick role.

Contextually, Mrs Sampson has no significant others while the residual mode relates to the fact that she had company while in hospital but was now alone in her flat.

Problem	Focal	Contextual	Residual
Behaviour Immobility Weakness	Pain in leg	Unable to get to the kitchen to cook for herself Constipated due to bad diet and immobility	Usually independent and now finds herself restricted
Anxiety Power- lessness	Fear of falling Unable to carry out activities of living	Pain prevents mobilisation	Loss of independence affects her self- confidence
Body image	Suffers from weight loss	Malnutrition and loneliness	Experiences change of body image which affects her self-concept

- health and illness are part of a continuum of life;
- the ability to adapt is defined by responses to stimuli;
- adaptive responses are zonal.

It is important to understand the nature of this classification and the fact that a number of concepts are identified as follows:

1. the nursing process/process of nursing and uses in practice;
2. the nature and scope of human behaviour and the way in which these impinge on responses to the environment;
3. the levels of assessment.

Modes of adaptation

Mode I

This is a *physiological* first-level assessment which deals with the activities of living (RENGLORS) as defined by:

*R*espiration
*E*xcretion
*N*utrition
*G*rowth
*L*ocomotion
*O*smoregulation
*R*eproduction
*S*ensitivity

The maintenance of homeostasis depends on the mutual working relationship of the different body systems and their interactions with each other. Thus the physiological mode relates to physical needs of the individual, such as exercise, rest, nutrition, fluid and electrolyte balance, and general maintenance of the internal environment within narrow limits for survival.

Mode II

This *Self-concept* mode relates to, and underpins, the way in which the individual sees himself in society. It includes the beliefs and feelings about self at a given time, formed particularly from perceptions of other reactions to internal and external environmental changes.

Mode III

This *role function* mode defines the sociological role played by the individual in society, e.g. a nurse, a parent, a teacher etc. It defines the expected behaviour that a person should perform to maintain a role in society.

Mode IV

This *interdependence* mode relates to a second level of assessment. It is in this mode that the individual relates to others and acknowledges the interdependency of human existence and actions. It is concerned with the comfortable balance between dependence and interdependence in relationship with others.

In conjunction with the above, there are two levels of assessment when caring for individuals with adaptive problems:

1. first-level assessment relates to the identification of the patient's maladaptive and ineffective behaviour;
2. second-level assessment identifies the stimuli or factors which influenced or underpinned the adaptive or maladaptive behaviour.

The nature of stimuli can be determined as defined by Roy as follows:

(a) Focal stimuli are those which confront the individual and require immediate response in order to maintain homeostasis. Thus in Mode I an acute infection results in immediate body reactions leading to hyperpyrexia and attempts to overcome the infecting micro-organisms.
(b) Contextual stimuli are contributory to the individual's adaptive responses to changes in the environment. Thus noise levels, environmental temperature changes and other external stimuli will affect the individual's response to changes and the context in which such a response takes place.
(c) residual stimuli are others not validated but nevertheless important in the assessment of responses to internal and external changes. These stimuli include activities arising from earlier experiences of the individual.

These stimuli are governed by two sets of processes in the body:

1. regulator, which is largely autonomic and are carried out by the nervous and endocrine systems in the body;
2. cognator, which is under conscious thought and involve individual decision-making.

20

The four modes define all aspects of assessment in the planning of nursing care. For example, Mode I represents the biological basis of nursing practice because it takes account of the physiological changes in the body. These changes reflect the dynamic relationships between the internal and external environments. Thus assessment in the nursing process covers this mode in which the biological integrity of the individual is assessed against a background of physiological functions.

On the other hand, Modes 2, 3 and 4 are essentially psychosocial and reflect interactions in these domains. The self-concept mode can reflect any of three views of the individual – personal, physical or interpersonal. Physically, the individual self-concept may relate to body functions and perceptions about normality, real or imagined, and the overall effect on personal well-being.

It must be noted, however, that the four modes are assessed together in order to obtain information about the whole person. The nursing process can therefore be derived from Roy's Adaptation Model as a holistic theoretical underpinning the implementation of care.

PROBLEMS OF HUMAN ADAPTATION

The ability to adapt is critical to human survival. The human organism must be adaptable because the internal environment must be kept relatively constant in spite of changes in the external environment. When homeostatic mechanisms fail, for whatever reasons, the ability to adapt successfully may be impaired. Thus in order to account for these factors, Roy suggests that physiological needs for homeostasis, self-concept, role function and interdependency should be considered by the nurse.

SUMMARY

A theory/model is a means to an end. Its purpose is to provide a framework for the planning of nursing and its systematic implementation. As can be seen from the introduction to the Roy Adaptation Model given in this chapter, it can be directly linked to the stages of the nursing process. It is, therefore, a practical framework for assessment, planning, implementation and evaluation of nursing care (Kim, 1983; Fraser, 1990).

REFERENCES

Fraser, M. (1990) *Using Conceptual Nursing in Practice* (Lippincott Nursing Series). London: Harper & Row.

Kim, H. S. (1983) *The Nature of Theoretical Thinking in Nursing*. Norwalk, Connecticut: Appleton-Century Croft.

Riehl, J. P. and Roy, C. (1980) *Conceptual Models for Nursing Practice*. Norwalk, Connecticut: Appleton-Century Croft.

Roper, N., Logan, W. and Tierney, A. (1990) *The Elements of Nursing, a Model for Nursing based on a Model for Living*, 3rd edn. Edinburgh: Churchill Livingstone.

CHAPTER THREE

Use of Roy Adaptation Model in practice
Justus Akinsanya

Contributors to this book will examine, in detail, Roy's Model in action, drawing on personal experiences as practitioners. In order to enable the reader to reinforce concepts and principles introduced, the following example is indicative of the type of nursing problems faced by individuals and the way in which the application of Roy's Model could assist the nurse to assess, plan, implement and evaluate nursing care.

Mrs Martin is a 23-year old with multiple sclerosis. She lives alone in a self-contained ground floor flat having recently been divorced from her husband who, unfortunately, felt overwhelmed and unable to continue with the marriage in view of the demands of caring for his wife. Mrs Martin was a secretary and had been married for five years. She had weakness of her lower limbs but manages her own cooking and other household work despite her disability. Mrs Martin needs help with physical care and support.

Using Roy's Adaptation Model, identify the nature of her nursing problems following admission to your ward.

From the information available on Mrs Martin, her reaction to the physiological mode (first level of assessment) will be as follows:

There are many sources for the collection of information on Mrs Martin. During the assessment part of her account, the nurse should use observational skills in relation to her own knowledge and experience in order to assess Mrs Martin's temperature, pulse and respiration. Her blood pressure should be taken and pressure areas examined with a view to generating a risk assessment score.

PHYSIOLOGICAL MODE

Having a marked weakness in her limbs and therefore a reduced mobility could lead to a number of potential health problems which would disrupt her normal physiological functions. Such problems include:

- constipation;
- incontinence;
- urinary infection;
- chest infection;
- dehydration;
- anorexia;
- malnutrition;
- insomnia;
- problems with personal hygiene;
- control of body temperature;
- psycho-social problems.

SELF-CONCEPT MODE

This is rather more complex and may be sensing a gradual physical loss in relation to her physical disabilities. She may well know that the marked weakness in her legs will deteriorate with time and, in view of her age and possible isolation, Mrs Martin will find the future daunting and frightening. Her sense of failure as a wife and prospective mother may also add to her feelings of powerlessness over her medical condition. Moreover, in a hospital where she is surrounded by able-bodied women of her own age group, she may become frustrated and appear to be unco-operative with nursing staff.

In order to promote positive adaptation, nurses looking after her will need to acknowledge Mrs Martin's abilities, where possible, and allow her the degree of independence commensurate with her prevailing physical condition. It would be important to identify her normal coping patterns and any variation in her present state should be documented. It is important that nurses assist Mrs Martin to identify her personal goals and to select actions to support a care

24

process for her if she is in state of disequilibrium on admission to the ward. When this has been established, efforts should then be made to plan her care to ensure self-help and autonomy while hospitalised.

It is important, throughout her stay in hospital and indeed after her discharge, that Mrs Martin should receive information on where to obtain help, e.g. from the community and social services. Her anxieties and perhaps feelings of guilt relating to her failed marriage and the trauma of having to cope with her disabilities alone, will require the services of a professional counsellor in order to improve her self-esteem and feelings of self-value and confidence.

ROLE FUNCTION MODE

It should be remembered that managing activities of living is a normal daily experience for every individual. Role functions within society are a reflection of individual psycho-social integrity and the expectations of the individual as a member of society. The performance of such a role will be affected by Mrs Martin's disabilities and her efforts to adapt to her changed circumstances would require professional support. Indeed, at every stage of life there are expectations concerning the performance, the growth and the development and behaviour appropriate to the individual's role in society. Although individuals can take on a multiplicity of roles, each role requires learning what is expected and the ways of acting to perform the role adequately.

This third mode of adaptation alerts us to the possibility of tensions which may arise when external demands upon a person's role performance fall outside the range of roles which the individual can accept. When she comes into hospital, Mrs Martin will have to take on the sick role and her independence will be threatened, with nursing staff having to do things for her which she should have done had she the physical ability to do them for herself. The need to take on a passive role in hospital would therefore reinforce her feelings of loss of independence.

INTERDEPENDENCE MODE

Interdependence, as we have seen, is the balance between the need to be independent and the dependent need to rely on others for attention and care. It covers the following aspects of adaptive responses: help seeking, attention seeking, affection seeking, obstacle mastery and taking initiatives. The aim of caring for Mrs Martin should be directed at helping her to adapt to the changing situation and to maintain a balance in her life. This would require her to relate to ward staff, other patients and the institutional environment in general. It is important that nurses caring for Mrs Martin identify the degree of her adaptive responses by assessing her problems and providing the appropriate professional support through nursing intervention.

Nursing intervention

It is important that no attempt should be made to 'take over' Mrs Martin's life while in hospital. She must be helped to maintain herself and to acquire and develop the ability to adapt to her physical conditions and the restrictions imposed on her by the changing bio-psycho-social situation. When the nurse does involve herself directly, it should be by following a careful assessment of Mrs Martin's needs and discussion of the areas in which she requires help in order to maintain her independence.

Some of the measures to be taken on admission and afterwards to ensure appropriate adaptive responses include:

1. introduction of staff and other patients to ensure social interaction;
2. explanations of medical and nursing actions;
3. maintenance of communication to establish short- and long-term goals;
4. provision of mechanical aids to enhance self-concept, role function and interdependency.

Mrs Martin's mental state should also be considered in the planning of her care. Thus her divorce may lead to feelings of rejection while the progressive nature of her condition may cause considerable anxiety to her. The use of Roy's Adaptation Model should therefore enable the nurse to take account of the diversity of factors which impinge on, and in the long term affect, the way in which Mrs Martin finally sees her conditions and the prospect of coping with her changed and changing circumstances.

CHAPTER FOUR

Applying the Model I
Lucy Fletcher

JUNE – THE INFORMAL CARER

This study attempts to explore and clarify some of the problems posed for a sick hospital patient who is herself the principal informal carer for a mentally disabled husband. Implicit in this exercise is an examination of the stresses experienced by informal carers in the community.

Much of this examination of Roy's model relates to the nursing assessment by Sister Saunders of Mrs June S, a 74 year old woman who has suffered a myocardial infarction. Crow (1979) argues that 'if insufficient time or trouble is taken over the assessment, fewer patient problems will be identified. This means that the second stage, that of constructing a care plan will not be as comprehensive as it might have been', with the logical conclusion that nursing care will be found to be deficient.

June was admitted to a Geriatric Assessment ward for observation and treatment, following a myocardial infarction suffered at home. Very shortly after her admission it became apparent that the nursing care she required involved an in-depth understanding of her social situation, principally because of her function as an informal carer.

She and Tom (her husband) were alone in the house and June was sitting in a chair one Sunday afternoon when she felt a severe pain across her chest. Momentarily, she 'blacked out' and was incontinent of urine. Once June recovered consciousness, she asked Tom to help her to bed, which he did. She then asked him to telephone the General Practitioner, to turn on the house lights and to open the front door. When the GP arrived he arranged for her immediate transfer to hospital, and also telephoned their daughter Mary, who met her parents on their arrival at the hospital. Tom was known by the psycho-geriatric services to be affected by dementia; his condition, however, has not resulted in in-patient treatment, and he is reviewed occasionally by a Community Psychiatric Nurse (CPN). June has coped well with him, showing tolerance and humour, and accepting only occasional help from their friends and neighbours – mainly to allow her to attend the Women's Institute meetings which are her principal source of social exchange and friendship.

Their daughter Mary lives locally, but only assists her mother when necessary and at her mother's request, and plays a fairly small part in the caring family situation as it existed on June's admission. June's care was the result of her deep love for her husband Tom, and one of her major expressed fears was that she should die first, leaving him alone in a world that was to him strange and hostile. Otherwise Tom was reasonably mobile and physically still fairly well, his mental condition manifesting itself as disorientation in time and place. His memory deficit was estimated at about 20 years, and he could be described as being late in Stage 1 of the three stages of Alzheimer's disease as described by Williams (1986).

When June and Tom arrived at the A&E Department, it was clear to the staff that Tom could not return home on his own, and Mary was unable to have him stay with her. No emergency Part 3 accommodation (Part 3 Accommodation is that outlined under the National Assistance Act 1948, and refers to the sheltered housing for the elderly staffed by Social Services personnel) could be found suitable for his psychiatric state, and so Tom was admitted to a ward that specialised in respite care. This allayed June's immediate fears over his future.

On arrival in the ward, June was not in any pain following administration of analgesia in the A&E Department. Following immediate care for her basic needs, and after checking her personal details, she was left to rest for a while. A basic care plan using Roper's model (Roper *et al.*, 1990) was then developed by an associate nurse to cover June's immediate physical needs. This care plan proved adequate for the very early period of admission, but on subsequent re-assessment, after June had rested, it was felt that it would not easily reflect her psychological and social needs. It therefore became imperative that another model should be selected.

Stevens (1984) aptly likens nursing theories and models to a map, where the use can pick out those parts that are important for any given purpose. Thus a nursing model can be regarded as a tool with which to improve the nursing care of a patient or client, the implication being that the model selected must reflect the needs of the individual rather than being imposed on all patients in the ward regardless of their needs.

The principal model of care to be considered and later adopted was Roy's Adaptation Model (Roy, 1970). Even the most cursory assessment had revealed that June's nursing needs were complex, and encompassed not only adaptation to the illness which she had suffered, but the cascade effect which that illness would have on her psychological and social functions.

Implementing the model: the first-level assessment

Blue *et al.* (1986) describe further major concepts developed by Roy, which extend understanding of the model. Adaptation can take place in four modes, the action of stressors leading potentially to maladaptation and a state of physical and mental ill-health. June's state of ill-health was initially within the physiological mode, but the major thrust of the nursing care requirements could be seen to fall within the disruption of the self-concept mode – her view of herself as a successful carer – with effects on role mastery, and interdependency modes since she had to that time needed only minimal help from Mary and others.

Role mastery, described by some writers as role function, was disrupted as June's infarct provoked a physical role failure. When Tom was admitted to hospital, June had to consider convalescence in order to regain sufficient fitness to function in her role as a carer. Interdependency in turn was affected, as the difficulties of maintaining a relationship with a demented spouse were highlighted by June's hospitalisation.

Within Roy's model a two-level assessment is indicated, with the first level describing the behaviours or symptoms displayed by the patient. Subsequently the nursing assessment continues to examine the stimuli, often described as stressors, which have brought about the behaviours. Nursing care planning and implementation are aimed at reducing, altering or balancing these stressors in order to return the behaviours to normal or near normal within a health-to-illness continuum.

Elimination

June stated that she found it very difficult indeed to use a bedpan and, until she was well enough to walk to the toilet, asked if she could use a commode by her bed instead. Normally she had no problems with elimination.

During her myocardial infarction June had sweated a lot and expressed a desire for a wash to 'freshen her up'.

Activity and rest

June stated that increasingly, as Tom had become more disorientated in time, she had lost more and more sleep at night and had become very tired as a result. Indeed at times she had found herself 'dropping off' during the day; as she still occasionally drove a car this development caused her a great deal of concern. Interestingly, Gaynor (1989) in a study of those who care at home for long-term neurological patients describes sleep loss as being a problem for informal carers at about month 28 after commencement of the caring role. June reported that Tom had become increasingly disturbed at night about 2 years prior to her admission.

Protection

Sato (1984) defines this category as skin integrity, however by using Andrews and Roy's (1986) 'protection', many other matters could be potentially included. For example, the nursing role in administration and monitoring of prescribed drug treatments as well as patient education in self-administration might gain entry to the first-level assessment, planning and implementation at this point. June stated that she was concerned at having to take coronary vaso-dilating drugs regularly, as she was worried that on her return home Tom might mistakenly take some.

June's skin was intact and her Norton score (Norton, 1975) of 15 placed her at low risk of developing pressure sores.

Senses

June had no auditory impairment, but needed glasses for reading, watching television and driving.

Fluids and electrolytes

June was not dehydrated on assessment. An intravenous catheter was in place, sited in the back of her right hand.

Neurological function

June was fully conscious and had been since her arrival on the ward. There were no complaints of pain although she described the chest pain she had experienced as 'crushing', and she is frightened that this pain might return. Mary considers her sleep deprivation as a definite stressor, Tom's increasing disability also worries June: 'How will I cope with him now'.

Endocrine function

June's blood sugar was within normal limits, and it was therefore unlikely that non-insulin dependent diabetes mellitus could be implicated in her myocardial infarction.

First-level assessment of the self-concept mode involves consideration of the patient's physical and psychological self-image. Price (1990) discussing self-image suggests that 'We should like to believe that our self-image is congruous with, and is an expression of, our personality. Yet we also guess that our self-image is strongly affected by what other people think of us. Self-image then is our own assessment of our social worth . . . . Self-image is important for our confidence, our motivation and our sense of achievement. As had already been shown in the physiological mode assessment, June identified definite stressors within this category as a result of her infarction. Despite the reliance placed on informal carers in the community, there is little public acclaim for the service that they provide. Therefore intrinsic self-image is liable to be severely disrupted by a disabling illness since the carer function is then affected. Extrinsic self-image (i.e. the public acknowledgement of the function of the carer) can also be seen to be damaged, as Tom had to be admitted to hospital for him to be adequately cared for in the absence of his wife. Both could potentially lead to feelings of low self-esteem and image on June's part.

The role function mode is examined within Roy's model as having primary, secondary and tertiary elements. The primary role is that descriptive biological role which is related to the person's age, physique and intelligence. The secondary roles are more complex, and have been interpreted by Nuwayhid (1984) as 'achieved positions, usually requiring specific role performance rather than qualities.' Further clarification is given in that 'secondary roles also imply a sense of stability in that they develop and are mastered over time, and are not easily relinquished.' June's caring role can be seen clearly to fall within this category. Tertiary roles are considered to be those often temporary roles associated with obligations and functions falling within the two previously described. Arguably June's membership of the Women's Institute, her principal recreation, which allowed her to function in her secondary role as carer and remain in reasonable psychological health within the primary elderly female role, comes in here.

June's roles can be represented as follows:

Primary role:	Elderly lady – prime support to husband Tom	
Secondary roles:		
Wife and carer to Tom	Mother to Mary and two sons who live away from home	Grandmother
Tertiary roles:	Member of the Women's Institute	Neighbour

The behaviours within the remaining mode to be assessed relate to those falling within the interdependence mode as conceptualised by Roy. Tedrow (1984) defines this as 'willingness and ability to love, respect and value others and to accept love, respect and value.' It has already been shown in this assessment that June's caring role arose from her deep love for her husband Tom, built on their years together prior to his dementia. It was clear that he too returned June's love despite his mental illness. This became clear when he absconded from the ward that he had been admitted to (on another site) and managed to catch a bus to the hospital where June was admitted. This would be comical – as well as a tribute to the lasting effects of bus route numbers – but for the fact that when he arrived and managed to locate June, his memory deficit proved unable to cope with the fact that his wife was an elderly lady. Tom had come to see a young woman, June 30 or so years ago, and could not recognise her. The effects of this incident were devastating to June, causing immense disruption within the interdependency mode and the primary nurse's role as counsellor came to the forefront as this problem developed. Within Roy's model, much of the nursing care devoted to psychological well-being is included as nurse–patient interactions take place.

It is a well known nursing phenomenon that people who are ill have increased needs for love, respect and affirmation from those surrounding them. As can be seen from this example, those caring for elderly demented people may experience traumatic upheavals when the partners are separated.

This examination, which has been expanded, completed the first-level assessment within the model. A summary is given below.

First-level Assessment	Patient: Mrs June S
PHYSIOLOGICAL MODE	
Oxygenation	Colour good, no cyanosis. Pale as a result of tiredness.
Nutrition	No allergies or special needs. Weight normal.
Elimination	States difficulty/discomfort in using bedpan. Skin uncomfortable due to sweating.
Activity and rest	Very tired. Recent tendency to 'drop off' at home.
Protection	Skin intact. Very worried about security of drugs once home because of Tom's poor mental state.
Senses	Auditory – no problems. Vision – glasses for close work.
Glucose and electrolytes	Hydrated. Intravenous catheter, (R) hand.
Neurological function	Conscious, no pain at present. Distressed by previous pain and feelings of inability to cope with Tom at present
Endocrine function	Blood Glucose 7.0/R No history of IDMM or NIDDM.
SELF-CONCEPT	
Intrinsic	Worries and anxious about her ability to manage Tom in the future: 'will it happen again?' Has coped well for many years with minimal outside help, although June states his

Extrinsic	condition is worsening and she is finding it difficult. Visits from Community Psychiatric Nurse only rarely, as not previously needed. No other services involved in support.
ROLE FUNCTION	
Primary	No disruption.
Secondary	Principal effects on role as caring wife. Difficulty in adapting to ill-health and patient role.
Tertiary	Unable to socialise during admission and while convalescent.

INTERDEPENDENCE

June describes her marriage to Tom as very happy. She appreciates that Tom's condition is affecting him emotionally and accepts this as part of his progressive condition.

Sister Saunders found that a short annotated style was practical in describing the behaviours outlined and allowed for a holistic picture of her patient's potential needs to appear. The process of obtaining the information was quite lengthy, but much could be learned from asking open questions evolving from June's own cues and by using a conversational style.

The second-level assessment

The second-level assessment relates to those behaviours observed in the first-level assessment and examines the three types of stimuli (stressors) which have caused maladaptation behaviours. Rambo (1984) considers that they need not be applied to all observed behaviours identified in the first level, but only to those leading to maladaptation.

In developing June's second-level assessment (see table) Sister Saunders found a difficulty. The myocardial infarction itself, described under the physiological mode, is a maladaptation that is possibly the result of stresses from both the ageing process in an elderly female and the stresses of caring for Tom. However, the myocardial infarction itself acted as the focal stress in examination of the self-concept changes, and the alterations in the role mastery and interdependence modes.

Second-level Assessment *Patient: Mrs June S*

Problem identified at first level	Focal stimulus	Contextual stimulus	Residual stimulus
PHYSIOLOGICAL MODE			
Elimination	Myocardial infarction	Difficulty using bedpan.	Privacy needed for elimination
Activity and rest	MI	Carer role resulting in loss of sleep.	self-value of caring role.
SELF-CONCEPT			
Intrinsic	MI	Has managed Tom well. Discusses feelings of low self-concept as MI has eroded her self-worth as carer.	Family value her as carer. June's mother cared for her parents.
Extrinsic	MI	Illness has resulted in husband's hospitalisation. June interested in possible other services available.	Society awards little praise to carers. Scarcity of services and respite for MI patients
ROLE FUNCTION	MI	(1) Difficulty in adapting to patient role and ill-health. (2) Loss of role as a carer. (3) Unable to socialise at present.	(1) Only previous admission was 30 years ago. (2) Values her effectiveness as a carer.
INTERDEPENDENCE	MI	Describes marriage as happy despite mental incapacity of husband.	Value placed by society on lasting happy marriage.

continued on page 36

table continued

Problem identified at first level	Focal stimulus	Contextual stimulus	Residual stimulus
Added later	MI	Tom unable to recognise June when visiting.	Poor understanding of Alzheimer's disease and its effects.

Examination of the stimuli

Focal stressors within the physiological mode. June's nursing needs, as revealed in the assessment of the physiological mode, are based on the behaviours both observed by Sister Saunders and reported by June in the first-level assessment. Those highlighted difficulty in using a bedpan, tiredness and worry about therapeutic drugs as matters related to her health disorder. Mercifully, her infarction proved to be relatively mild despite its potentially serious nature.

Contextual stimuli within the psychological mode were more difficult to identify, although June's age and the physiological effects of prolonged stress can be assumed. Drugs fall within the category of contextual stimuli – especially since drugs which may alter either behaviours or psychological function include the hypotensive and coronary vasodilators that June was prescribed.

However, June's clearly identified concern regarding the safety of her medication on her return home makes this a matter for nursing concern. Ways and means of preventing Tom mistakenly taking her drugs had to be explored to reduce June's anxiety on this score. Eventually a secure pack was found to be suitable, and arrangements were made by the pharmacy to supply these to her.

Residual stimuli are those relating to the values and experiences owned by the individual. June's only other admission to hospital had been some 30 years before; perhaps that is where Tom's misconceptions arose. The implications though are that the enormous changes that have taken place in the nursing care and management of acutely ill people may result in misconceptions, particularly those involving the shift from medical models of care to the nursing-orientated direction taken today. June enjoyed being a partner in the evolution of care although there is some current evidence that this is not always the case (Waterworth and Luker, 1990).

Throughout the self-concept, role function and interdependence modes, the focal stressor is the physical illness itself, which resulted in the highlighting of previously undetected problems relating to June's function as a carer.

Serious difficulties have arisen within the self-concept mode as shown in the assessment. June's own value of herself as a carer was affected (shown as intrinsic self-concept). Thus this became a vital part of her nursing needs, as her feelings towards her perceived failure in her expectations of herself produced a loss of confidence and fear for her future self-esteem.

Extrinsic self-concept, interpreted as the way in which society by and large ignores informal carers until a crisis emerges, was also highlighted: June, discussing the matter felt that she was being a nuisance and 'causing problems'. The question must be asked, should a carer feel guilt in this situation? Nolan and Grant (1989), reviewing the situation of informal carers, describe how they should have the right to time off for themselves, to be consulted in policy matters, to have priority in some services, training for their caring role, availability of counselling, and to be able to choose the model of care best suited to their needs. In addition, the literature describes how, if carer stress is to be prevented, emotional support is a vital need.

Role function (role mastery) can also be seen to be eroded by the myocardial infarction acting as a focal stimulus or stressor. Physical role failure within the secondary roles of wife, mother and grandmother can be clearly seen. Disruption within the self-concept, as outlined, may also produce a ripple effect should depression develop and a vicious cycle begin, as the self-concept and self-esteem become poorer and result in further physical role failure. It should also be reiterated that June had not been in hospital for many years, thus she had to adapt and accept to some extent the new role of patient forced upon her by circumstances.

Fear of dying first was one of June's most clearly expressed worries: 'what would happen to Tom if I died first'. She acknowledged that Tom could not cope alone, as clearly demonstrated by his admission to hospital. The myocardial infarction caused her to examine the possibilities of long-term care for her husband and she and her family contacted a number of care settings with a view to planning for Tom's long-term future.

June's undoubted role-mastery within her secondary role as a carer was also completely altered by her illness. Not only did nursing care face the challenge of helping her to adapt to this change, but also to liaise with social workers and her family to arrange a period of convalescence to allow her to recover fully.

Interdependence. It should be emphasised that this was added to the assessment later as the need arose. As discussed previously, June and Tom had had a very close relationship throughout their marriage. Initially June felt little change had occurred as a result of her illness and the admission of both herself and Tom to hospital care. As described earlier, this happy state received a rude shock when Tom arrived unexpectedly on the ward. Contextual stimulus therefore arose in this mode as Tom's mental incapacity became startlingly evident. June was very distressed by Tom's non-recognition of her and considerable length of time was spent with her in helping overcome her upset.

Planning the care. As mentioned earlier, June's myocardial infarction needed little intervention apart from coronary vaso-dilating drugs. It has not been necessary within this study to detail the care needed by a patient who has suffered from this condition. Nursing needs proved very simple. For instance, her preference for using a commode rather than a bedpan and her need for rest required none of the 'high-tech' care usually considered necessary following myocardial infarction.

June's nursing care as identified in the assessment related almost entirely to those psycho-social needs associated with her role as a carer. Here it should be stressed that non-verbal communication is also a vital component, the use of comforting touch and non-threatening body language being a part of the care given.

June's need for counselling was paramount if the disturbance in her self-concept was to be overcome and her needs within the role mastery and interdependence modes met. Here the difficulties of counselling a patient in a busy ward became apparent. Privacy, one of the prime factors in successful counselling, was difficult to achieve at least until June was considered medically fit enough to be taken to a quiet room in a wheelchair. Confidentiality had also to be maintained, creating some problems in evaluating the successes or difficulties arising from counselling. Recording these on the care plan had to rely on the referrals to other agencies, with handover being principally verbal using a case conference approach in order that June could have the maximum support from all the nursing team.

Logan (1990) states 'For the Roy Model to be compatible with the current interpretation of accurate nursing diagnosis statements, stimuli must be amenable to independent nurse functions'. June's illness was medically uncomplicated, however nursing care came into its own in meeting her needs for counselling and understanding the disruption in her life that had occurred. The use of Roy's model allowed these needs to be quantified, highlighted and a counselling approach adopted. The success of the model was demonstrated when the nursing data were used to prolong her admission to hospital until she was able to attend a convalescent centre. The date were quantified by the model and used to argue the case when the consultant geriatrician reviewed June's case. The model also outlined some specific needs that could be met by outside agencies once she and Tom returned home, with a view hopefully to supporting her and reducing the stresses of caring for Tom. The nursing role in co-ordinating these services within the care of the elderly is a vital skill within the speciality.

Some caution however, must be exercised as the nurse interprets the data obtained while assessing the self-concept, role mastery and interdependence modes. Data obtained within the physiological mode and the focal stimuli are necessarily objective, as facts are being reported. This may not be the case when the other three modes are assessed, and the nurse's own perceptions, values and culture can affect the findings. June is an elderly English lady from what is broadly known as the middle classes and a similar background to Sister Saunders who developed the assessment and care plan. While this is open to misunderstanding, that potential must be magnified when care plans for those of different class, tradition and culture are being developed.

Study guide

1. While on clinical placement, talk to three informal (i.e. unpaid) carers. Discuss with them separately the positive and negative aspects of caring for a physical or mentally dependent person. Assess what might cause them stress, both physical and mental.
2. While working in the community, discuss with community workers what support is available to informal carers in the area where you are working.
3. Using Roy's concepts of primary, secondary and tertiary roles, draw up an assessment box like the one applying to June (page 32). What are your own roles?

4. In a small group, discuss how the counselling process can be adapted and used in patient care within the general hospital:

   (a) Where might counselling take place in privacy?
   (b) How can confidentiality be maintained?

   Use the UKCC Code of Conduct for reference.

PAUL – OVERDOSE OF PARACETAMOL WITH ALCOHOL

Paul arrived on the ward, semi-conscious, having taken an overdose of paracetamol with alcohol. He had been initially treated in the Accident and Emergency Department and an intravenous infusion of acetylcysteine (Parvolex) in 5% dextrose was in progress. Paul's notes gave the information that he had probably taken the overdose about 6 hours previously, and that he had been found by his landlord.

Intentional self-poisoning is on the increase within the UK (Jones, 1977; McMurray et al., 1987; Wynne et al., 1987). This appears to be the situation also in Europe as work by Danish and Dutch researchers (Ott et al., 1990; Kienhorst et al., 1990) demonstrates. Paracetamol is a mild analgesic, easily available in large quantities from chemists, and is often implicated in suicidal or parasuicidal self-poisoning among young people. Older persons are considered more likely to take other drugs, perhaps a reflection of a more complex medical history resulting in a greater number of prescription-only drugs being taken. It was not possible for the Accident and Emergency staff to establish how much of the drug had been taken, only that an empty 50 tablet bottle had been found in the living room of Paul's flat.

Paul was 20 years old and single, currently living in a small rented flat. His appearance was unkempt, with long hair which did not appear to have been washed recently and he had not shaved for some days. His clothing was grubby. There was nobody accompanying him to the ward, and his Accident and Emergency notes recorded his next of kin as his mother who lived some 200 miles away. The landlord had called the ambulance and supplied the crew with what little he knew of Paul's background, including the fact that Paul was unemployed. It became significant to Paul's care that during his admission to hospital there were no telephone calls enquiring about his welfare and that his only visitors were an old friend of his and his friend's mother.

In this study, Roy's model of nursing is used as a framework to describe the care needed by this patient – a young man who no longer wished to live and who could see no way out of his difficulties. The study considers the assessment and planning phases of the model, and necessarily includes some reflection on the role of the nurse within the situation examined. The nature of Paul's admission limits this study to the acute phases of his recovery from an overdose and his subsequent transfer to the Mental Health Unit. It follows also that the principal emphasis in the care planning relates to the physiological mode.

Assessment

An accurate assessment is a logical and essential step in the delivery of good nursing care. Mental Health patients, under which heading Paul could be broadly classified, were identified as long ago as 1972 by Stockwell in her classic research *The Unpopular Patient* as being a less favoured group of clients within the acute medical setting. Assessing patients within this category requires patience and empathy if a thorough and workable plan of care is to be constructed and an evaluation of that care developed. Only then can the nurse reflect on the effectiveness of the nursing care delivered and potentially audit for quality of care. On several models of nursing being used on the ward at the time, Roy's model (Roy, 1984) was selected by Staff Nurse Julie, the named nurse in Paul's care. By the use of Roy's model, a holistic picture can be developed and care delivered accordingly. Roy's model became a particularly attractive framework for Paul when it became known that his admission period would extend from the Thursday afternoon of his admission until at least Tuesday of the following week as a result of two factors. Firstly, no Psychiatric Out Patients appointment would be available before that date. Secondly, the Acute Mental Health nursing unit had no bed available and was reluctant to admit Paul anyway until his physical symptoms were stable. This gave Julie time to assess Paul in depth and plan his care.

Gathering data in order to develop the assessment proved to be a fairly lengthy process, as initially Paul was drowsy and incoherent owing to the effects of the alcohol and the paracetamol. Because of his state, Julie merely confirmed his details as given by Accident and Emergency, maintained Paul's safety by close observation and care of his IVI and allowed Paul to rest and sleep for a while.

Despite the fact that Paul could be roused, he did have some essential safety needs. The ingestion of alcohol and consequent irritation of the gastric mucosa result in nausea, with a risk of vomiting during which the vomitus can easily be inhaled with dire results for a semi-conscious patient. His intravenous infusion of acetylcysteine in 5% dextrose was acting as an antidote to the hepatotoxic effects of the paracetamol and required careful regulation if the therapeutic effects of the drug were to continue.

Gradually Paul regained consciousness, and full assessment of his nursing needs became possible during the evening of his admission. Julie did however start to develop her first-level assessment before Paul became full conscious. This is in line with Roy's own description of the first-level assessment as 'The Nurse looks at the person's responses, internal or external, that can be observed or measured, or which are subjectivity reported.' Some subjective inferences could also be made from Paul's appearance: he was unkempt, with greasy hair and dirty skin, and his clothing which had been sent with him from A&E was soiled, worn and grubby. Physically he was thin. As he came round, Paul was adamant that he wished to be left alone, expressed suicidal thoughts and said that he had hoped to die as there was nothing left. The fact that he was expressing these thoughts to Julie allowed her to question him gently about why he felt that way. Paul's parents had been divorced when Paul was 10, and he felt that his father had rejected him and his mother. There was no longer any contact, even though Paul had written to him when he became engaged to his girlfriend Kate. These previously unexpressed feelings of rejection had been increased when Paul's mother had asked him to leave home two years ago. Paul had rented a bedsit, and continued his job in a factory. He then met Kate and eventually they took the tenancy of the small flat in which Paul now lived. Both partners were working and all was going well in both his relationship with Kate and in his job. The factory then closed, leaving Paul unemployed. Kate continued paying the rent from her earnings and Paul was in receipt of unemployment benefit but with only poor job prospects. The relationship became strained and about two weeks earlier Kate had left the flat, and broken off their engagement. Paul had difficulty in obtaining housing benefit and was finding it hard to manage paying the bills and keeping up the flat. He admitted to not eating much and then only poor food. Indeed he said that he had not eaten for some days and in an effort to 'cheer himself up' had bought half a bottle of whisky with his dole money. It was as he drank this that he became extremely depressed and had taken the paracetamol.

Identifying the focal contextual and residual stimuli in Paul's care proved challenging. Taking an overdose of paracetamol with alcohol proved dramatically that he was unable to cope and adapt to negative influences and stressors within his life and could be described as an extreme example of maladaptation. Firm identification of the prime focal stimulus which caused Paul to take his overdose was difficult and can be argued to be the cumulative result of many problems. His feelings of rejection by his parents and by Kate, the loss of his job and his poor financial state all played a contributory part. In addition he was also required to adapt to an environment – the ward – whose aims of preserving his life were dramatically opposed to his own – ending it – thus even as his physiological needs were met, further stresses arose.

The focal stimuli proved difficult to identify, as discussed, and consideration of the contextual and residual stimuli potentially brought into question a conflict between the internal factors left by Paul and those of the nurse's own feelings. It is important here to stress that Paul had been admitted to a general medical ward where the skilled support that he needed from the mental health team was not available.

Please now turn to the review questions at the end of this chapter.

Planning Paul's care

The immediate care plan was based on the first- and second-level assessments within the physiological mode. As described, Paul arrived on the ward semi-conscious, although able to be roused, and incoherent from the effects of alcohol. So the assessment and care plan had to be grounded firmly in the observed behaviours of the first level of assessment.

Essentially this care plan revolved around Paul's safety needs and the prevention of long-term complications from the drug overdose. Some of the objectives were necessarily short term until Paul was conscious and able to meet his own internal and external safety needs.

Not all the headings within the RENGLORS mnemonic needed to be planned, but Paul exhibited maladaptive behaviours and potential maladaptations under Respiration, Nutrition, Osmoregulation and Sensitivity:

PHYSIOLOGICAL MODE	
Respiration	Paul will be safely positioned in order to prevent his airway becoming obstructed by vomitus (from ingestion of alcohol and paracetamol). REVIEW CONSTANTLY UNTIL CAN BE ROUSED.
Nutrition	Vomitus to be cleared immediately to prevent reinforcement of feelings of poor self-esteem and helplessness. REVIEW 8 HOURS.
Osmoregulation	Infusion to be monitored to preserve maximum therapeutic effect. REVIEW 6 HOURS.
Sensitivity	(a) Semi-conscious but can be roused. Observe for deepening of unconscious state. (b) Use of touch to prevent feelings of isolation and develop caring communication. GOALS: (i) REVIEW 8 hours. (ii) 24 hours to facilitate communication.

The other three modes all showed disruption and maladaptive behaviours and Julie was able to plan Paul's care in more detail relating to these modes the following day. By then Paul was able to communicate more freely despite what he described as a 'dreadful' hangover. Planning care to meet his needs in the three more psychological modes required enormous empathy from Julie. It is perhaps this demand on the nurse-delivering care that renders caring for the self-harming patient on a general ward so unpopular. Depression and anguish at the loss of a role and relationship with accompanying poor self-esteem is not an uncommon life experience through which many have lived or have imagined. It is easy therefore not only to cease to view the patient and his care objectively but to recall the nurse's own experiences and own developed values in this situation.

Prior to commencing her assessment of the self-concept, role function and interdependence modes, Julie added two more items to the physiological care plan:

```
PHYSIOLOGICAL MODE
Sensitivity              Headache/pain caused by the inges-
                         tion of alcohol:
                         • NO ANALGESIA TO BE GIVEN
                           DUE TO POTENTIAL LIVER
                           DAMAGE
                         (this was also entered on Paul's pre-
                         scription chart).
                         To encourage oral fluids.
                         Allow Paul to seek a quiet place on
                         the ward.
                         To orientate Paul to the ward, there-
                         by facilitating communication levels
                         with other staff and patients. REVIEW
                         8 HOURS.
```

Paul decided that he would like to sit in a corner of the day room. This allowed Julie to care for her other patients and then return to Paul at a time when conversation could be conducted in an unhurried manner. During the conversation, planning of care was discussed as Paul expressed what he would like to do and how he felt about his perceived problems.

The other problem added to Paul's physiological assessment related to the potential after-effects of an overdose of paracetamol. Paul was unable to recall how many tablets he had taken and so he was assumed to have taken the full bottle of 50 tablets, in order to provide a margin of safety. The maximum toxic effects of paracetamol develop about 4 days after ingestion (British National Formulary, 1992) with the patient becoming more confused and showing deepening loss of consciousness as a result of hepatic encephalopathy. The outcome is usually fatal. Research conducted by Gazzard *et al.*, (1976) suggests that young people overdosing on paracetamol have no knowledge of this delayed effect, and indeed would not have chosen the drug had they known of the delay between return of consciousness after the initial overdose and the onset of these serious symptoms. The last problem to be added to Paul's physiological plan reflected the more long-term dangers to Paul's physiological equilibrium.

PHYSIOLOGICAL MODE	
Sensitivity	Potential problem, as a result of overdose: observe for altering conscious state and confusion. Report any changes immediately to medical staff. REVIEW: ON-GOING.

Some of Paul's care plan in the three psychological areas related to his physical appearance. Paul's background as a trainee manager suggested to Julie that he might, when in normal health, appreciate a smart appearance which in turn might elevate his mood and possibly reduce his poor self-concept:

SELF-CONCEPT	
Poor self-worth	Reinforced by unkempt appearance. Paul agrees to bath and shave during the afternoon. Contact friend Graham (tel: 123456) who will collect clothes from the flat and bring them to the ward. Paul to wear his own clothes when clean clothing is available. Soiled clothing placed in bag. Paul to be allowed to verbalise his views of himself to encourage free communication. Non-judgemental nursing approach. • PAUL AGREES NOT TO LEAVE WARD WITHOUT SPEAKING TO STAFF FIRST (potential suicide risk). PLEASE ACCOMPANY PAUL IF HE WISHES TO LEAVE WARD. REVIEW DAILY.
ROLE FUNCTION Unemployed male	Previously management trainee in local factory. Financial difficulties.

> Paul encouraged to discuss his
> feelings about the loss of his
> job, and other interests which
> could lead to employment.
> Agrees to see social worker re-
> garding his financial situation.
> Referral sent (date).

Discussing Paul's job loss did prove difficult for Julie because of his alienation. Paul saw her as 'well, you are one of them aren't you. YOU have a nice secure job in nursing'. It emerged that Paul had been thought of as one of the brighter recruits to his firm, and had been expected to go a long way. He had rejected the opportunity of higher education in favour of earning a living and becoming truly independent. It was these feelings that proved almost insurmountable for him, and all that could be done in the general ward setting was to allow him to express his negative views and try to reinforce any positive thoughts. It would be impossible for the hospital to meet his needs, of which the primary one was paid employment at a level which was to him acceptable (i.e. where he had left off).

Paul had also experienced prolonged disruption in his interdependence needs, that is those needs for belonging, interrelationships with others, love and affection. As discussed at the beginning of this chapter, Paul's parents had divorced when he was 10 and his father had recently rejected his advances when Paul wrote to him about Kate. Paul's mother had asked him to leave her home when he was 18, which Paul blamed on her new relationship. Subsequently she had left the area to be with her new partner. During his hospital admission, Paul requested that she should not be told of his overdose. The breakdown of his engagement to Kate acted as the last straw and Paul commented 'That was it, nobody wanted me, or cared . . . I had no parents to turn to, no girlfriend, not even a job to go to where I was useful'. The only person he felt he could turn to now was his friend Graham, with whom he had gone to school and who remained a close friend. When Julie suggested that Paul would feel better in himself if he had some clean clothes to wear, it was Graham that he suggested could go to the flat to collect them. Julie telephoned Graham who was happy to do so. Later on that day (the second of Paul's admission) Graham visited the ward and spent some time talking to his friend. Graham's mother was willing to wash his old and soiled clothes and sent in some of his favourite food (macaroni cheese) which could be reheated in the ward microwave.

INTERDEPENDENCE NEEDS

Expressions of rejection	Contributory factors: parents' divorce, mother moved away, breakdown of loving relationship.
	Paul to be allowed to express his views, and verbalise his feelings about his relationship breakdown.
	Friend Graham contacted (see self-esteem).
	Graham to be encouraged to visit.
	Paul shown how to use the ward telephone so he could contact Graham. Graham's mother has supplied change for the phone.
	Reinforce that the provision of food (the macaroni cheese) was a physical expression of care and the provision of comfort.
	REVIEW DAILY/ONGOING.

Outcome of Paul's admission

Paul's assessment and care planning did not prove to be an easy task for Julie. Care within the physiological mode was relatively straightforward, demanding a knowledge of the physiological aspects of the after-effects of paracetamol overdose. Julie made sure that the other members of the ward team were fully aware of the potential risks so that all could play a part in observing his progress and notify any improvement to her, or dramatic deterioration to the medical staff immediately.

As discussed within this study, Julie was able to assess the maladaptive behaviours arising within the self-concept mode using a physical model based on the observation of his behaviours in the first level of assessment. However, these physical manifestations arose within the cognator domain, as described in Chapter 2, and intervention at the physical level on evaluating care did have an effect on Paul's psychological deficit. By allowing Paul to verbalise his views of himself, insight could be gained which allowed Julie to assess disruption in the other two modes more realistically.

Communication was handicapped in the role function mode. As discussed, Paul viewed Julie as being on the other side of a divide, the employed and the unemployed, with the expectation on his part that those in employment would have no understanding of the plight of those without jobs. Employment is regarded by many as fulfilling not only a role but answering the needs for belonging and esteem that are necessary to psychological well-being. Additionally, the traditional male bread-winner role is threatened by unemployment. As Paul had done well in his job, viewed it as having a long-term future and was well regarded by his manager, the loss of his job was devastating to him and played a large contributory part in his subsequent overdose. He was able to express much of these feelings but always allied to the expressions of 'them and us' which would render empathy on both sides difficult because of his alienation. About his interdependence needs, Paul was frank that he was not worth loving or caring about, and although his mood did improve during his admission he still demonstrated considerable maladaptation in this area.

Paul was admitted to the ward on a Thursday afternoon, and attended a Psychiatric Out Patient Clinic on the Tuesday morning. It was decided that his mental health was sufficiently affected to warrant admission to the Mental Health Unit attached to the hospital, which he did so as a voluntary patient. Julie, when evaluating his care and the use of the model, felt that although many of his needs remained unmet at the time of his transfer, skilled nursing in the Mental Health Unit would continue and consolidate the work she had started on the general medical ward. To assist in this aim, his general nursing notes were transferred with him.

Postscript

Paul did recover from this most stressful period in his life. He decided to apply for a degree course and is now attending university, where he has a good social life. He hopes that at the end of his course his employment prospects will be enhanced.

Review questions

1. A suicide attempt is perhaps the archetypal maladaptation response. Paul faced numerous stressors, each of which was interpreted and given meaning through his cognitive activity (cognator function). To what extent do you think Paul's critical situation was brought about by:

   (a) focal and contextual stressors,
   (b) residual stressors,
   (c) cognitive functions (his interpretation of events and their meaning for his life)?

2. Paul's circumstances throw up the point that each individual has a limited capacity to adapt. One of the key roles for health care professionals is health education, and by implication healthy adaptive responses. What might these be, and to what extent can general nursing contribute towards them?

3. Paul found himself on a ward more used to physical care than the delivery of mental health care support. The nurses were unclear on how to tackle the first- and second-level assessment of Paul's role function or his interdependence modes. What might result if care is delivered primarily in one mode?

4. How might the nurse usefully and tactfully explain the delayed effects of the paracetamol overdose upon Paul's liver to him? (Remember there are issues of informed consent and the impact of uncertainly to be dealt with here!)

5. Patients who have taken an overdose are fairly routinely admitted to hospital wards. Spend a few minutes considering your own attitudes towards this group of patients.

Exercise

One of the problems contributing to Paul's maladaptation was his lack of financial resources. This is clearly demonstrated by his alienation along a dividing line of those who are employed and have no worries and those who are not employed and have insufficient financial resources for successful adaptation. In order to develop your understanding of people in this situation ascertain:

What is the rate of unemployment benefit and how is it paid to the recipient?
Which agency pays housing benefit and what factors influence its payment?

REFERENCES

For June

Andrews, H. and Roy, C. (1986) *Essentials of the Roy Adaptation Model.* Englewood Cliffs, New Jersey: Prentice-Hall.

Blue, C. L. *et al.* (1986) Sr. Callista Roy – Adaptation Model. In Marriner, A., *Nursing Theorists and their Work.* St Louis, Missouri: Mosby.

Crow, J. (1979) Assessment. In Kratz, C., *The Nursing Process.* London: Ballière Tindall.

Gaynor, S. (1989) When the caregiver becomes the patient. *Geriatric Nursing,* May/June, 120–123.

Logan, M. (1990) The Roy Adaptation Model: are nursing diagnoses amenable to independent nurse functions? *Journal of Advanced Nursing,* **15**, 468–470.

Nolan, M. and Grant, G. (1989) Addressing the needs of informal carers: a neglected area of nursing practice. *Journal of Advanced Nursing,* **14,** 950–961.

Norton, D. (1975) Research on the problems of pressure sores. *Nursing Mirror,* **140**(7), 65–67.

Nuwayhid, K. A. (1984) Role function theory. In Roy, C., *Introduction to Nursing, an Adaptation Model,* 2nd edn. Englewood Cliffs, New Jersey: Prentice-Hall.

Price, B. (1990) Body image. In *Nursing Concepts and Care.* Englewood Cliffs, New Jersey: Prentice-Hall.

Rambo, B. (1984) *Adaptation Nursing, Assessment and Intervention.* New York: Saunders.

Roper, N., Logan, W. and Tierney, A. (1990) *The Elements of Nursing, a Model for Nursing based on a Model of Living,* 3rd edn. Edinburgh: Churchill Livingstone.

Roy, C. (1970) Adaptation, a conceptual framework for nursing. *Nursing Outlook,* **19**(4), 42.

Sato, M. K. (1984) Skin integrity. In Roy, C., *Introduction to Nursing, an Adaptation Model,* 2nd edn. Englewood Cliffs, New Jersey: Prentice-Hall.

Stevens, B. (1984) *Nursing Theory: Analysis, Application and Evaluation.* Boston, Massachusetts: Little, Brown.

Tedrow, M. P. (1984) Interdependence: theory and development. In Roy, C., *Introduction to Nursing, an Adaptation Model,* 2nd edn. Englewood Cliffs, New Jersey: Prentice-Hall.

Waterworth, S. and Luker, K. (1990) Reluctant collaborators: do patients want to be involved in decisions concerning care? *Journal of Advanced Nursing,* **15**, 971–976.

Williams, L. (1986) Alzheimers: the need for caring. *Journal of Gerontological Nursing,* **12**(2), 21–27.

For Paul

British National Formulary (1992) No. 24 (September), p 18. London: British Medical Association and Royal Pharmaceutical Society of Great Britain.

Gazzard, B. *et al.* (1976) Why do people use paracetamol for suicide? *British Medical Journal,* **1**(6003), 212–213.

Jones, D. I. (1977) Self poisoning with drugs; the past 20 years in Sheffield. *British Medical Journal,* **1**(6052), 28–29.

Kienhorst, C. *et al.* (1990) Characteristics of suicide attempters in a population based on a sample of Dutch adolescents. *British Journal of Psychiatry,* **156,** 243–248.

McMurray, J. *et al.* (1987) Trends in analgesic self poisoning in West Fife 1971–1985. *Quarterly Journal of Medicine,* **65**(246), 835–843.

Ott, P. *et al.* (1990) Consumption, overdose and death from analgesics during a period of over the counter availability of paracetamol in Denmark. *Journal of Internal Medicine,* **227**(6), 423–428.

Roy, C. (1984) *Introduction to Nursing, an Adaptation Model,* 2nd edn. p 46. Englewood Cliffs, New Jersey: Prentice-Hall.

Stockwell, F. (1972) *The Unpopular Patient.* London: Royal College of Nursing.

Wynne, H. *et al.* (1987) Age and self-poisoning; the epidemiology in Newcastle upon Tyne in the 1980's. *Human Toxicology,* **6**(6), 511–515.

CHAPTER FIVE

Applying the Model II
Carol Crouch

ROY'S MODEL – A BASIS FOR A HELPING RELATIONSHIP

We need to adapt to many new circumstances and situations during our lives. As people we need to adapt to life events such as getting older, changes in our family or working situations or changes in our own and friends' and relatives' health status. In fact any change in our way of living as people requires us to adapt.

This chapter describes adaptation to a normal life event – Moira's fourth pregnancy. Moira is a college lecturer aged 36, and this pregnancy presented new stimuli in the form of many new challenges for her. Circumstances that were different for Moira during this pregnancy from her earlier ones were: her husband Donald's decision to become self-employed and the developmental stages of her other children.

This care study examines how Laura, Moira's health visitor, established a helping relationship with her using Roy's model as a framework. Although this chapter was intended to illustrate the formulation of a first- and second-level assessment, it also clearly demonstrates the extent to which steps of the nursing process are interlinked in practice. While in the process of compiling the assessment, Laura needs to reflect in an evaluative sense and also begin to work actively with Moira, the client, thus using the implementation step of the process. We will focus on Laura's thoughts and reflections as she strives to understand how Moira views her individual world. Roy's model is used as a framework for arranging and building these ideas into an assessment.

Moira is a busy college lecturer, married to Donald, who has just started her own business. Moira and Donald have three children:

53

Mary, aged 12 and the eldest, Patrick who is nearly 10 and Declan who is 2. Laura's first meeting with Moira was during the ante-natal clinic at Moira's GP surgery. Laura has found that meeting clients before the baby is born enables her to begin the assessment process. This first meeting was to establish contact with Moira and to find out how she felt about her pregnancy and the way she was adapting to her situation.

Moira describes how she is feeling . . . 'I am managing . . . and I feel very well. Donald is away quite a lot but he helps at the week-ends. It was Donald who wanted another child he thought it would be good for Declan'.

Laura has found that it is not helpful to ask a list of questions, so she listened attentively noting who and what Moira talked about and the way that she did this. 'This baby was planned so that he or she would be born at the beginning of the holidays: I have until September to get things organised . . . It is important for me to work: I feel I am a better mother because I work . . . and we are hoping to employ a nanny who will look after Declan as well as the new one . . .'. Moira went on to say that she saw herself as well organised and relied on Donald's help when he was at home.

Laura was aware of the adaptation problems which a busy working mother needs to cope with. She also knew that marital equality as far as the home and domestic chores were concerned did not happen in reality (Henwood, 1987) and most of the responsibility was shouldered by the woman.

Moira went on to describe Declan's birth and the pain she described as the worst pain she had experienced. Moira continued 'I do not like being fat: I think it's because I cannot take any exercise . . . I know that pregnancy doesn't stop you but I have had some stress incontinence; I continued to play badminton but I sometimes have to leave the court; needing the loo in the middle of a game . . . I do the exercises when I remember'.

On reflection, Laura thought that Moira was actively adapting to her situation in a positive way but wondered if Moira also felt some conflict and ambivalence about her pregnancy. Moira was concerned about the birth: she feared it would be painful and she would not be able to cope. It was also apparent that Moira did not want to say any more about her fears about the pain. She had changed the subject, and Laura had respected her wish not to dwell on the expected pain.

Assessment of the physiological mode was not attempted as Moira's ante-natal care was at the moment being supervised by the community midwife and her GP. The meeting was purely to begin to form a relationship between health visitor and client, and also for Laura to begin to understand what this infant would mean to Moira and her family.

Laura did not offer any advice or pose any searching questions during this interview. The skills used in collating a nursing assessment are those of observation, interviewing and measuring (Tierney, 1984). The nurse, in addition to these skills, needs to identify with the human experience (Morse, 1992). It is this ability to appreciate and identify with another person's humanity that increases our effectiveness as nurses. An accurate and detailed nursing assessment is important because without it care planning will not be accurate, individual or patient centred (Price, 1987; Thompson, 1990).

Roy and Andrews (1991) describe a two-level assessment. In the first level, the nurse assesses the client or patient behaviours in each adaptive mode. The second-level assessment requires the nurse to assess the stimuli which influence the behaviour in each adaptive mode. Roy and Andrews (1991) suggest we adapt and cope with our lives by responding to stimuli in each adaptive mode. Our adaptation to any event or situation depends on several factors such as the degree to which the perceived stimuli or stresses are affecting our life. The stronger the stresses are felt, the more impetus those stimuli provide for adaptation. These 'strong stimuli' are the focal stimuli, that is the stimulus of stresses which are so powerful that they cannot be ignored.

Whatever happens to us is always associated with other factors, that is to say it is always in context. This associated factor Roy and Andrews (1991) call the contextual stimuli. Stresses and stimuli also have some background or foundation, which are the residual stimuli. The residual stimuli may be seen as the factors in our lives which have settled down out of sight, in a similar way to chalk settling in a glass of water. If this settled residue or residual substance is stirred or shaken up, it bubbles to the surface. The residual stimuli bubble to the surface in a similar way and then become contextual or focal. When the residual stimuli are verbalised by the patient they become contextual or focal. Stimuli change in emphasis with time. What will be a focal stimulus at one time may change to contextual at another.

The residual stimuli may also be theoretical or experimental knowledge understood by the nurse but not by the patient. This knowledge will influence and guide the nurse in making assumptions or hypotheses in order to plan nursing care.

Adaptation takes place in two ways and Roy and Andrews (1991) describe them as regulator and cognator. Both forms of adaptation require abilities and preparation. Without some form of foundation, adaptation would be like diverting a train along a route without any track.

Regulator adaptation, such as drinking in response to thirst, requires a functioning hormonal and nervous system. Without this network we would not be able to regulate our fluid intake and output. In the same way our cognator function needs a foundation of realisation, awareness and the skills and desire to change behaviour before adaptation can be achieved. This network is formed by our perception, past experience and learning.

Laura's main concern was to understand how Moira was adapting to this particular life event. So she concentrated on assessing Moira's behaviours in the self-concept, role function and interdependence modes. Assessment of behaviour will be followed by the factors influencing those behaviours, the stimuli or stressors. The type of stimuli will be indicated by: F – focal stimuli; C – contextual stimuli, and R – residual stimuli.

Before we start to summarise Moira's behaviours we need to consider the significance and importance of *self-concept*. Self-concept can be simply described as 'how we think of ourselves', but behind this frequently used term lies all the complex issues of our identity and therefore our thoughts, feelings and attitudes about ourselves. The self-concept mode focuses on the psycho-spiritual aspects of the person.

Roy and Andrews (1991) describe the basic need underlying our self-concept as psychic integrity. Adaptation in this mode is to strive for a sense of equilibrium in maintaining a sense of 'who am I'.

In order for the nurse to appreciate the whole person, understanding self-concept is crucial. The person as an integral whole is a combination of a physical self and a personal self. First the *physical self*: this sub-heading is used to assess how we view the body and the vehicle of our existence, and this includes our body sensation and image.

The *personal self* is a little more complex: this includes concepts such as *self-consistency*. We all try and maintain a sense of stability or equilibrium in how we ideally like to be viewed by ourselves and others. Finally, personal self includes the *moral* and *ethical* and the *self-ideal* aspects of our lives – the values and beliefs we have about ourselves. Basically the moral–ethical–spiritual self is about personal values, rules and principles that are considered important to us as an individual. This is part of our self-esteem, our feelings of value and worth. Self-ideal is how we would like to be, to ourselves and others.

The value that we have about ourselves may affect our ability to adapt, and in some instances inhibit physical and or psychic healing.

The concept of self and who we are as a person is psychologically and philosophically complex. Roy's self-concept mode is based on the work of many theorists, and these are described in detail on page 272 of her book *The Roy Adaptation Model, the Definitive Statement* (Roy and Andrews, 1991).

Summary of Moira's behaviour in self-concept mode

Physical self or body sensation: Moira said she did not like being fat, and she talked about being fat with distaste.

Considering that she was an active independent woman, it was strange that Moira had not regularly organised and completed the pelvic floor exercises. Laura felt that this behaviour, which seemed uncharacteristic, demonstrated some ambivalence, perhaps about the pregnancy.

Personal self: self-ideal

Laura felt she learnt most about Moira's idea of herself from her non-verbal behaviour. She had looked at Laura steadily while speaking and had spoken in a confident and self-assured manner. When she had talked she had shown a serious attitude to health care, parenting and her work. This seriousness led Laura to hypothesise that Moira had a tough and rigorous specification for herself.

Self-consistency

Moira wanted to be organised and in control of her life.

Moral–ethical–spiritual self

Moira had high expectations and standards for herself and possibly for others.

Assessment of stimuli, influencing self-concept mode; focal (F), contextual (C), residual (R)

Pregnancy and lack of exercise made Moira feel unattractive (F).

She needed to be an organised person and her life was about to be disrupted (C).

Stress incontinence meant Moira could not exercise. Her husband Donald was supportive and helped physically but did not organise (C).

Moira needed to be in control and had high expectations of herself

(R). Roy and Andrews (1991) describe the residual stimuli as the factors that influence the situation but which are only alluded to or are unclear. The effects of the residual stimuli are not confirmed.

Summary of behaviours in role mastery

Moira's primary role as an adult woman was one that she viewed seriously – she acted responsibly and was self-sufficient. Secondary roles for Moira were as a wife, mother and lecturer. She had spoken in a concerned and caring way about the children and Donald.

Roy and Andrews (1991) suggest that problems in role mastery usually arise in secondary roles. Laura knew from her own experience as a working mother how difficult it was to give enough energy to each of these important roles. Moira had emphasised the role of lecturer and had shown that her role as a 'good mother' was to an extent dependent on her work. Laura noted the reference to the 'good mother' and speculated about this being another indication of Moira's ideal self.

Tertiary roles were not assessed. Laura was aware that Moira had referred to playing badminton but she had not mentioned any other outside interests.

Summary of stimuli influencing role mastery

Moira needed to be organised (F). She had high standards for herself and needed to be a 'good' mother and lecturer (C). Moira is tired and needs energy to cope with pregnancy and work (C).

As a working mother Moira did not have an informal peer support network, such as mother and toddler groups or contact with other mothers (R).

Summary of behaviours in interdependence mode

Moira needed to be or feel independent in adapting to her new family situations (F). She needed and liked Donald's help but he was working away during the week (C). Moira liked to manage her own problem-solving (C). Moira's self-sufficient attitude may be a response to negative experience with health professionals (R).

This brief meeting provided Laura with an important start to both the assessment and their working relationship. Their next meeting would be eleven days after the birth of the baby.

It was a bright sunny day for Laura's first visit to Moira's home. When Laura arrived, Moira was feeding the baby in the garden.

Walking through the house Moira observed the safety gate across the stairs and the guard in front of the gas fire. The hall and the room leading to the garden were littered with toys and Declan was riding his bike around the garden. Laura wanted to ask many questions about the birth and how Moira was managing, but she has found that letting the clients tell their own story helps her to gain valuable contextual knowledge about them and how they see their world.

Moira settled herself down and continued to breast feed the baby. 'The birth wasn't as bad as I had expected, she was lighter than Declan and it was much easier. I was only in hospital for three hours'. Moira went on to describe how she and Donald had managed the 'labour' and how she had found the clary sage and lavender massage helpful. She also admitted to 'sneaking in' clary sage and lavender into the bath at the hospital.

Donald had worked at home the first week and had helped with the children and looked after her. She did not have any other help as her parents were dead and Donald's parents lived abroad. She went on to say how difficult she was finding Mary's behaviour but refused Laura's offer to discuss it. She changed the subject and went on to say the baby was called Nula and how concerned she was about Nula's feeding. 'She seems to need feeding all the time, she is not a happy baby. That also concerns me because I think contentment is important because I believe that patterns established in infancy influence later life. I have always had contented babies . . ., the baby harness helps . . ., but because she wants to feed all the time my nipples become sore'.

She went on to describe how upset she was about the red rash on Nula's face. She thought it looked awful and upset her because she wanted her baby to be beautiful. Moira had spoken to her GP about the spots, who diagnosed a staphylococcal infection and had prescribed a course of antibiotics.

Laura asked Moira if she could see how Nula was feeding and moved her chair so that she could see clearly. Watching Moira feed Laura could see that Nula had not got sufficient breast areolar tissue in her mouth. She explained to Moira, 'some babies just do not open their mouths wide enough, which means they latch on to just the nipple, and this leads to the soreness'. She also recommended that Moira could try holding Nula in a different position when feeding Nula, which would help to deal with the soreness (Royal College of Midwives, 1991). Laura asked Moira to let her know if the problem continued, as she could refer Moira to the breast feeding counsellor. When Moira continued, Laura changed the subject. 'The midwife reminded me before she left about contraception. Now this is worrying; I have been thinking about it'. Moira studied Laura's face and carried on. 'The best type of contraception for us is the coil', she continued. 'Declan was born after eight years and I had a coil then, ... we had not planned to have any more children after Pat ... I must make an appointment at the family planning clinic'.

This meeting confirmed for Laura how independent Moira was. Moira had looked in a rather shocked way when Laura had asked to see how she was feeding. Laura was not put off by this, since although Moira had breast fed three babies each one is different. She also wondered if Moira had in the past had a negative experience with health professionals. This might account for the attitude of 'I can manage'. As Laura felt this attitude might interfere with their working relationship she decided to discuss it with Moira. Moira told Laura how she felt that she needed to battle with health professionals in order to be heard and have her wishes acknowledged. She had not felt she had a good relationship with the midwife whom she thought had ridiculed some of her ideas. Laura remembered reading about health professionals who use a traditional approach (Foster and Mayall, 1990). Using this approach, health workers have a pre-conceived idea of how clients should behave. The professional health workers, having defined a criterion, urged the client to change their behaviour to fit this idea or ideal. Laura assured Moira that in her experience it was important for individuals to define their own difficulties and then actively explore alternative solutions. She also hoped Moira would see her as a facilitator or partner rather than as someone who would tell her what to do – that is as someone who could help her to explore issues.

Self-concept

Moira was returning to what she thought was a reasonable size; it also seemed that her attractiveness and size were linked in some way. Laura thought Moira seemed to be comfortable with her sexuality. She continued breast feeding in a natural and composed way, and talked about her sexuality and contraception in the same manner. She was mainly concerned about Nula. Laura had been surprised at Moira's remark about wanting Nula to be beautiful. She had assumed that this would not be so important to Moira who appeared so sensible. Moira had talked about her sexual relationship in an easy and relaxed manner. But she had been insistent about what she considered to be the only satisfactory method of contraception. The comment and the admission of 'sneaking' in the oils helped to confirm for Laura the concern of Moira about trusting health professionals.

Assessment of stimuli affecting self-concept mode

Moira felt that it was her responsibility to organise the contraception (F). Moira may have expected value judgements about her feeling that having a coil inserted was the best form of contraception for her. This in turn led to her being insistent in the way she told Laura about it (C). Past experience for Moira of using the coil was that she became pregnant. This would make her nervous and apprehensive about relying on it (R).

Nula's discontent threatened Moira's perception of herself as a 'good mother' and her ideal self of wanting everything to be organised like 'a well oiled system'. Laura could not decide if Moira's ideal self was a residual or a contextual stimulus. She was not sure to what extent Moira recognised and was aware of that aspect of herself and how it affected her behaviour. Laura could now perceive the less logical and more emotional aspect of Moira's personality. For instance, wanting her baby to be beautiful and insisting the coil was the only method of contraception which would suit them.

Assessment of behaviours in role mastery mode

During this meeting Moira had not mentioned her job at the polytechnic. She appeared to be immersed in the family and integrating the new baby into her life. The baby's discontent was distressing to Moira, and she felt Nula's unhappiness was a reflection on her parenting. There was also the reference to Mary and the quick assertion that 'Mary would come round'. Laura felt that it was important for Moira to do things in her own way. Laura also felt that too active an intervention from her would be unwelcome. She needed to gain Moira's trust and then Moira would ask for help if she needed it. Adaptation for Moira appeared energetic and active but Laura wondered if Moira's adaptation was as positive as it appeared. She did not want to talk about Mary and she also had admitted her reluctance to trust health professionals. Laura reflected on the direct way that she had talked about the contraception and the way that Moira had anticipated the enquiry about sex. Laura was also aware of Moira's enquiring mind and positive way of dealing with situations, for example, the use of essential oils and massage during the labour might mean that Moira may feel that she *should* be able to manage or that she *ought* to get everything right.

Assessment of stimuli influencing Moira's role function

For Moira, Nula's need to feed constantly and her discontentment was worrying (F). The spots on Nula's face were also a sign that all was not 'beautiful' with the new baby (F).

Moira said constant feeding was causing sore nipples. She lacked knowledge about the cause of sore nipples (C), but might refuse to see the breast feeding counsellor. These difficulties might reflect on Moira's view of herself as a parent (R).

Moira's intellectual and emotional self may be in conflict (R). Mary was 'being difficult' and this could mean she was becoming another discontented child (C).

Moira firmly believed that it was important for infants to be happy. She thought that contentment was important for serenity and a happy adult life. Contented and 'good' babies are thought to be happy babies, so it could be argued that this idea is a cultural 'norm' and a commonly held belief about the importance of childhood experiences and how they influence future development (C). Moira feels it is her responsibility to provide a serene and solicitous environment (R).

Assessment of behaviour in interdependence mode

Laura still had a strong impression that Moira did not want help and feared that she (Laura) might interfere or contradict her ideas in some way. Conversely Laura admired the way Moira was managing to adapt to a demanding situation but was concerned about the 'keep out' signal which was continually flagged up.

Assessment of stimuli influencing Moira's interdependence mode

Moira needed to be or to feel independent (F). She needed to be in control of her life and decide who she needed to help her, for example, family planning for contraception, the GP for Nula's spots (C).

Her situation had changed which meant she needed to adapt or adjust her relationships. Laura wondered if anyone had told Moira how capable and effective she was. Moira needed Donald's approval but perhaps he rarely verbalised what he thought (R). A lack of peer or family support might contribute to Moira's independent attitude (R).

Parenting is a secondary role and Moira was actively coping with this. That was demonstrated by behaviours such as speaking to her GP and Laura. She was talking about her concerns and seeking a solution. Laura felt that Moira was not able to talk about her relationship with Mary in the same way. Laura noted that the stimulus concerning Nula was contextual, but with Mary it was residual. Laura felt Moira's independence and 'high standards' for herself prevented her from discussing Mary with Laura. Laura also knew Moira would need to trust her before talking about important emotional or difficult issues.

Moira was coping effectively with her concern about contraception; she had articulated her concern and had resolved to seek expert help. Laura felt the lack of harmony in terms of Nula and Mary was a considerable stress for Moira.

Ten days later Moira brought Nula to the clinic because she was still worried about the rash on Nula's face. The prescribed antibiotic had been ineffective. Moira asked Laura if she thought it might be eczema or a heat rash. The 'rash' was across Nula's nose, spreading across her cheeks and top lip. Nula's nose had papular spots on it which looked weepy and sore. She also had nappy rash. Laura thought that the rash did not look like a heart rash or eczema but recommended that Moira consult the clinic paediatrician and ask her opinion. Laura promised to see Moira after the consultation.

Following the interview with the clinic doctor Moira looked angry and upset. 'She said that she didn't think it was a staphylococcal infection', and as Moira said this she nodded towards the surgery door. 'At last I felt that someone was interested and was taking notice of what I said. As the spots have been there since shortly after she was born the doctor started asking me about my health at the end of my pregnancy . . . and I remembered that I had vaginal thrush shortly before she was born. The thrush cleared up quickly so I didn't think any more about it. I do remember when I was pregnant with Pat that thrush was quite a problem. I have got some cream to put on Nula's face. So we will see . . . at least it seems to be making sense now and I am glad you said to come if I was worried'. Laura and Moira went on to discuss if Moira could think of any other ways that Nula might be passified. She said she had considered an orthodontic dummy and perhaps she would try one.

Laura asked about Moira's nipples:

'They are still sore and one is cracked, I have started to treat it with an essential oil which has antiseptic properties... I have a friend who is an aromatherapist. I tried changing the way I held her when feeding but she did not like it, so that did not work'.

Laura apologised to Moira for overlooking the possibility that Nula might have thrush. Thrush and the resulting sore mouth are often the reason for babies not sucking vigorously; then they are hungry and unhappy, which makes them demand feeding frequently (Royal College of Midwives, 1991).

Laura did not reflect on this interview for several days but when she did she remembered Moira's relief about the 'rash', at least there seemed to be some logic and basis for the diagnosis of a fungus infection. Laura respected Moira's wish to try an essential oil for her nipples and she wondered if the oil and the cream would work.

The following week Laura made a home visit. Nula was now twenty four days old. Moira was working marking some exam scripts and Nula was sleeping in her pram in the garden. The situation was a little better for Moira; the rash on Nula's bottom and face had improved. The dummy did satisfy her need to suck continually and Moira felt the oil had helped her sore nipples.

Laura asked Moira if an added pressure was the high standards she set for herself and others. Moira's reply was a rather ambiguous 'perhaps'. 'I am trying to get some work done, reading the scripts and marking isn't too bad but I need to write some reports and I am not finding time to do them, I am exhausted after a day of coping with her and Declan. I feel I have to be on guard all the time when he is around as I am never sure what he will do next'. 'Still it is early days yet', she said brightly but added looking glum 'I hate feeling so tired..., it is also difficult when Declan is here, because he is so young he has to be watched constantly, and it means I have precious little time to myself. I so look forward to Donald being home at the weekends'.

Laura was aware that Moira was thinking about work again. She also reflected on Moira's dismissal of having high ideals for herself. Laura knew from her experience that clients would often think about what was said in their own time and then discuss it when they were ready.

Laura's next visit was about two weeks later. Moira had not visited the clinic or been to see her GP so Laura hoped this meant that life was easier for Moira and that Nula was settling.

This visit was during the school summer holidays. Patrick (Moira's eldest son) was painting at an easel with Declan, and a girl who

Laura thought must be Mary rushed past Laura and disappeared upstairs. Moira began by apologising for Mary's behaviour. 'I am sorry she appeared so rude ... nothing seems to be right. She is particularly resentful of the time I spend with Declan ... but it's easier now the holidays have started'. She rushed over to stop Declan from tipping paint into Nula's pram, asked Pat to watch what Declan was doing for a short time and then sat down again. 'Mary is usually better when I can give her some time, we seem to rub each other up the wrong way, she is so volatile and so argumentative'. She laughed and continued, 'I suppose I want everything to be smooth and easy ...'.

Laura asked Moira to consider how realistic it was to expect that life could be agreeable for everyone with no fighting or jealousy. Moira looked contemplative for a short while and then looked at Laura: 'the person you want to hear about is Nula isn't it ... well I know of course that you are interested in all the children. Nula's fine now, she still takes a long time to settle and is sometimes niggly, but since her face and bottom cleared up she is much better ... not as contented as I would like but ... I have thought about my expectations of myself'. Moira's voice faded here as if she didn't want to finish.

'I went to the family planning clinic, where I saw a very pleasant woman who patiently answered all my questions ... they make the coils from copper instead of plastic now, and they are more reliable. She also reassured me by saying it would be unlikely that I would be in the 2% failure again ...'. 'How are you coping with that?' 'Mmm well I am not going to think too much about that, I suppose sterilisation would be an option ... I really don't want any more children'. She went over to pick Nula up who had started to cry. 'I am pleased to have got it sorted out, and they were most helpful ... there are two things that I have got to get sorted now, one is our holiday and the other a nanny. I will organise the nanny when we come back. We are away for three weeks in total and I will have six weeks when I get back before term starts'. Laura arranged to visit again in four weeks' time.

Moira's view of herself as an organised and capable person was still challenged by Nula not being a contented baby and also by Mary's 'argumentativeness'.

Laura thought, as Moira had mentioned her expectations of herself, that this might mean the stimuli had changed from residual to contextual. Parenting for women does seem to centre on the home environment. Women are traditionally responsible for the emotional and physical environment of the family. The work of the male is still seen as employment and therefore outside of the home (Henwood, 1987).

Sorting out the contraception and reconciling the idea of the coil appeared to be a relief to Moira. She saw the whole issue of the contraception as her responsibility.

Towards the end of the summer Laura was aware that Moira would be busy organising herself and the children in order to return to work. Laura made an appointment to see her at home. On the day Laura called Moira had arranged for Jane, the new nanny, to take the children out. She went on to say Jane seemed rather young. 'I thought it would be a good idea if she started before I went back to college. I am more concerned about how she will cope with Declan, I don't want him to spend all day watching TV. When he was with the child minder there were other children and she organised activities for them all. I want him to have plenty of stimulating activities and I wondered if I should make out a schedule for him. What do you think?'

'Making out a weekly routine of activities may also help Jane to organise herself,' Laura agreed. 'Yes I will say it is just a guide rather than a set programme but I will also say that I think he should only watch TV once a day, either in the morning or the afternoon'. 'You seem to be happy that Jane will cope with Nula'.

'I was upset about stopping breast feeding. I know you said I could do both, bottle and breast feed, but I prefer to do it this way. It was rather a battle, well not a battle but as with the dummy she didn't like the texture of the teats . . .'. Moira looked pensive for a moment and went on giggling to herself. 'She isn't what I would call a contented baby and she does take a while to settle, and for some reason it was more difficult at night. My breasts still feel as if they are filling when she cries and especially at night. However I found that she took the bottle at night from Donald and settled when he fed her. When he is away she would cry and refuse the bottle. I suddenly thought she can smell me or my milk'. She chuckled gleefully, 'do you know what I do now? When Donald is away and I have to feed her I put Donald's mac over my nightie. It works. I hold her against his coat and she takes it like a lamb. Would you believe it . . . but I do feel sad that I am not feeding her any more. Having said that, I know that I am a more tolerant and calm person when I am working'.

Laura thought it was important to tell Moira how well she had managed. Each new child needed to be integrated into the family, which inevitably meant disruption. It was this disturbance which Moira found unpleasant. Moira then told Laura that she did not see herself as capable or as a good parent, and she needed to be in control to help her lack of confidence.

Assessment of stimuli affecting Moira's self-concept

Moira needed to be in control and would have liked to view herself as a calm, contented, capable person (F). She also knew that in order to achieve this she needed to have the stimulation and satisfaction of her job (C).

Past experience may have contributed to Moira's negative view of herself (R). She possibly had hoped to organise the family and emotional aspects of her life with the same efficiency that she applied to her job.

Assessment of role function behaviour

Moira's important roles were linked with her self-concept. The family were important to her but she also needed a role outside the home. Her work helped her to achieve her ideal of being a good mother and therefore of having a harmonious and happy family.

Assessment of stimuli affecting role mastery

Moira needed to excel in all of her roles – mother, wife and lecturer (F). She did not like asking for help (C). She found health care professionals judgemental (C).

Assessment of behaviour in interdependent mode

Although Moira would describe herself as an independent person, she was dependent on others for help and support. Donald's help and approval were of paramount importance. She was now going to depend on Jane. Although she would influence how she cared for the children, Moira would need to rely on Jane being punctual and capable. It could also be argued that Moira was dependent on her work as a college lecturer as this was such an important aspect of her life. Perhaps Moira's need to be in control and manage by herself prevented her from establishing helping relationships quickly.

Assessment of stimuli influencing interdependent mode

There were now new demands in Moira's life. Moira's previous experience of parenting was not useful for this new child (F). Moira liked to find her own direction and did not like relying on other people (C).

Adaptation

Attempts to change are often sabotaged by our usual habitual behaviour. We all have usual ways of coping and dealing with the situations confronting us. These ways are usually well-established patterns of behaviour that previous experience has helped to refine and master. Changing well-established ideas or behaviours requires a concentrated, sustained effort. If the concentration slips then the old patterns take over. Moira had accepted the responsibility for organising the domestic aspects of her family life.

This sense of responsibility made her fiercely independent and insular. She had a firmly held belief that her children's future happiness depended on a contented childhood. The communications media disseminate this view of the 'good mother' to all parents. The ideal of the always smiling, totally tolerant parent increases the stress and stimuli on parents. Conversely, children need to be confronted and helped to deal with adversity in order to learn to adapt (Winnicot, 1986). This belief and ideal placed demands and stresses on Moira, and Laura suspected that she was reluctant to risk changing this ideal.

In order to conclude this assessment, Laura reflected on how the concepts which make up Roy's model helped her understanding of Moira.

Health visiting is hard to define (Cawley, 1991), and most health visitors would not describe themselves as nurses. They would say that they were concerned with health education and in helping people develop their parenting skills, but they are still concerned with caring. It is important for the health visitor, or any teacher come to that, to understand the client's concerns in the way in which the client sees them. They must recognise who is important to the client and what matters most in the client's life. Laura thought she did understand how important it was for Moira to be in control and find her own solutions.

Laura communicated this to her by asking her to think of other ways of coping, for example, she could have suggested a dummy, but instead asked Moira to think of alternatives. When Moira was concerned about the coil, Laura simply made the statement that it seemed important. Moira was able to do the rest.

Laura suspected that Moira's experience with health professionals had been difficult, because she did seem to expect Laura to contradict her or insist that her way was best. It was necessary to confront this and change this aspect of stimuli from residual to contextual. Once it was acknowledged it became easier to be honest with Moira. Laura could then list alternatives for Moira and then she could choose what she would like to try.

Laura was cross with herself for not thinking about thrush, but she felt her apology was an important step. Not assuming the role of the all-knowing expert was a good start for building a relationship. Mothers will often feel more relaxed in talking about their difficulties to professionals if they can see professionals acknowledge their own strengths and weaknesses – what Morse (1992) calls 'our humanity'.

Laura was unsure if she should have been more challenging about Moira's relationship with Mary. She felt that Moira's ideal self did not want to confront this issue of jealousy and rivalry. Laura was fairly sure that Moira would deal with this issue should it become a 'focal stimulus'. Laura hoped that Moira would see her (Laura) as a resource should the situation become more urgent.

Laura found the concepts of Roy's model useful because she felt she was quickly able to understand what Moira thought about herself and her body. Assessing behaviours and stimuli in the self-concept mode helped her to reflect and to see Moira as she saw herself.

Laura found that she could now appreciate that there is often conflict within each of the modes, and life was a sort of balancing act. For instance, Moira had planned the pregnancy but hated being fat. She saw herself as an energetic, busy, well-organised person but the tiredness she felt when she was breast feeding and looking after Declan was difficult for her. Laura reflected and questioned if she should have asked Moira how much sleep and rest she was getting. Laura felt there was considerable conflict for Moira in the *role mastery mode*.

The family was important to her but she also valued and enjoyed her work. Laura did wonder if Moira wanted to apply the organisational skills that she used at work to managing the family. Laura considered whether she could have made it easier for Moira to talk about her feelings.

Laura thought that the assessment structure was helpful – each mode interrelated with the other so the whole person was always in view. Laura felt it was important to remember that one aspect of the self affects another part of the person. For instance, Moira's ideal self was a calm, serene, understanding and patient mother, but in order to achieve this she felt that she needed to work. Then this need to work brought her into conflict with the other side of parenting, that is to do everything and create and control a harmonious environment for her children.

Adaptation occasionally means changing well-established patterns of behaviour and the adaptation level depends on the stimuli; for example, Moira needed to arrange a method of contraception. The need to deal with this was the focal stimulus, however she did not want to think about the residual stimulus of 2% failure rate. Laura felt her main task was to recognise and to perceive Moira as a person and how she coped with life changes so she could use her as a resource if she wanted to. Her task was not only to make judgements about effective and ineffective responses but to set up an effective communication network based on a sound framework. The judgements about ineffective or effective coping could then be made by Moira herself. Communication is the linchpin of all nursing and caring, and without this all efforts and action would be unproductive (Benner and Wrubel, 1989).

Questions

1. Moira's assessment concentrated on self-concept, role mastery and interdependence. In which mode do you think Moira found adaptation easiest? Which do you think was the most difficult?
2. The skills used in assessment are described as observation, interviewing and measuring. Which of these skills did Laura use and when?
3. How well do you think Laura achieved her ideal of being a facilitator and partner?
4. To what extent do you think Laura was able to establish a helping relationship with Moira?
5. Identify the factors which you feel contributed to a helping relationship and those which hindered.
6. Do you think Laura should have challenged Moira about her attitude to Mary? If you do, how would you have initiated this?

Activity

The activity for this chapter is a fantasy role play. This fantasy exercise is designed to help you gain an insight into the body and role changes that pregnancy may cause. This activity will also help you to appreciate how individual an experience self-concept, role function and interdependence are.

This activity is a guided fantasy and is concerned with pregnancy and child birth. A guided fantasy is a useful way of experiencing a situation or an event by imagining what it might be like. It does require you to relax and allow yourself to be influenced by the script.

The description of the experience needs to be made as real as possible by your imagination. So if you are told that it is dark and quiet, you must conjure up just that in your mind's eye. It is also important to have a sense of how it might feel if you were sitting somewhere dark and quiet.

The feelings are subjective and each person will have a different experience of the fantasy. Sharing these experiences in a group is a useful way of learning and accepting how different people feel about situations and consequently how they then react.

Any person dealing with issues related to this topic may want to opt out. For example, if you or a close friend or partner have been treated for infertility or have experienced a still birth, abortion or miscarriage, this may be a difficult experience.

The script has been written so that the fantasy can be used for both men and women.

Equipment required

- Tape recorder
- Tape of soothing, relaxing music (I use Barber's *Adagio for Strings)*
- In a group situation, a quiet comfortable room is important

This exercise may be completed by an individual. The text can be read into a tape recorder to make a tape of instructions and background music. This can then be played back. Before the exercise, have to hand a pad and pen so that your feelings and responses can be recorded.

Start by sitting or lying comfortably, with a sheet of paper and a pen nearby. Close your eyes and clear your mind of the concerns of the day. Imagine in your mind something smooth and dark – sheets of soft black velvet, or a dark clear sky.

Concentrate on your breathing – breathe with rhythm. Take a breath in and imagine that breath going into your lungs down to the bottom of your chest, and then breathe out.

Breathe in . . . and then out, . . .
Breathe in . . . and then out . . .
Breathe in through your nose, fill your chest . . . and out through your mouth . . .
Breathe in through your nose, fill your chest . . . and out through your mouth

The script

The first change you notice is the tiredness and feeling of being upset inside. Your body feels abused, tired and strained, and you ache inside.

The tiredness is rather like being druggged and not being able to shake it off, to stay awake. The delicate digestion is more of a nuisance, the only thing that seems to settle it is eating.

This has started a pattern of comfort eating. Eating starchy bland food helps to settle and tranquillise the delicate feelings in your stomach.

You have started to put on weight, clothes do not fit, and the only ones you can wear are shapeless and large. The weight and fatness are accompanied by slowness and a feeling of being bloated. Your abdomen particularly feels heavy and large, and there are problems with your bladder. Several times you have only just managed to get to the loo in time. You are now continuously afraid that you are not going to make it in time.

The huge bloated abdomen also causes heartburn. This burning sensation starts after most meals and is particularly unpleasant at night.

Sleep is disturbed by this indigestion or heartburn and by having to wake up to turn over. You have consciously to manoeuvre yourself around the bed to turn over. This contributes to your tiredness. It is dark and cold when the pain starts. There is a dragging sensation in the pelvis and the groins. Walking around helps you at this stage, and you find sitting in a warm bath soothing.

Gripping pain sweeps over the whole of your abdomen, and there is also a sharp pain in your back at the bottom of your spine. You are aware that the pains are fairly constant and you are becoming exhausted.

As exhaustion levels go, this could be compared with a long steep hill climb, leaving you breathless and sweating with an aching head from the effort involved. It is all such hard work and exhausting.

You are given a small frail infant. This tiny, fragile being will only survive if you care for it and keep it safe. The appealing, rather minute creature needs constant attention. Being so small it cannot eat large meals, and so needs food at regular, short intervals. The food needs to be of a special type, warm and especially clean.

The infant's skin is delicate and sensitive, and needs attention such as creaming or oiling to prevent it from becoming sore.

This small person does sleep but the sleep pattern does not coincide with yours. Frequently you just fall asleep and this dependent, small person wails for attention.

You cannot go too far away in case it needs anything. You feel guilty if you decide to ignore the wailing and get on with what you are doing.

You are responsible for this small person's start in life: for health in terms of nourishment and clean food; well-being in relation to comfort stimulation and safety. Survival is dependent on being kept out of danger. Another small life is relying on you knowing the right things and also doing the right things.

Now, write on a piece of paper the answers to the following questions:

1. How do you feel about yourself?
2. How do you feel about your change in body size?
3. How would your life change, taking on this full-time caring role?
4. How do you feel about this small person's dependency on you?
5. How much would you manage to keep a sense of your own identity?
6. How do you view your role as principle carer and protector?

In order to de-role and leave the fantasy, imagine yourself walking along a long, straight road. There are trees on either side which block your view of the surrounding countryside.

At the end of the road you see the room in which you are sitting or lying. Look at the room, remember where you are and what the day is. Say what day it is out loud. Also, repeat your name and something about yourself, for example, 'I am Camille, and I am cooking spaghetti for supper tonight'. Such a statement will help to establish reality and de-roling from the fantasy.

CHRISTINE – A STUDY IN INTERDEPENDENCE

This care study describes how Rachel, a community nurse, used Roy's Model as a framework of adaptation for Christine who was terminally ill. The purpose of this care study is to demonstrate how Roy's Model helped Rachel the community nurse to understand Christine's needs, her care, her death, and to question could she have done more. Christine was described by Rachel as enigmatic and a deeper level of understanding of Christine as a person was only possible for Rachel after Christine had died. Rachel felt that she had helped Christine to adapt to her illness but only in a limited way. She felt care of Christine had been mostly reactive and had concentrated on her physical needs.

Rachel felt that Christine's adaptation was mainly to deal with her physical discomforts. Christine did not or could not discuss her emotional or psychological needs. In order to make sense and take stock, reason and reflect, Rachel used Roy's concept of adaptation in evaluating how effectively she felt Christine had adapted and coped with her illness, dying and death.

Christine

Christine's medical diagnosis of carcinoma of the lung was made two years ago. She had remained well following surgery and radiotherapy until three weeks ago when she experienced difficulty in swallowing and recurrent bouts of unproductive coughing. Christine's GP was advised by the radiotherapist responsible for Christine's care that further active treatment was not possible and that Christine had asked to be discharged as she wanted to be at home.

Christine had lived for all of her 36 years in the same house with her parents. Her sister who was four years older was married and lived 20 miles away. Christine had remained living at home and each weekday commuted into London where she worked as a legal secretary. Most of her adult life she had been a help and solace to her father during her mother's frequent and long hospital admissions for depression. Her mother had recently been discharged following negotiations between Dr Bennett (the family's GP) and the psychiatrist responsible for her mother. Christine's mother had been told of Christine's illness but her father did not want her to be told of the severity or the prognosis of the illness.

Evaluation

Evaluation is often described as the last step in the nursing process. Evaluation is important for the nurse because, as we have already described, in order to learn about patient care we need continuously to evaluate not only the models used in a theoretical sense but our skills in applying them in practice. This care study provides an opportunity for a detailed retrospective examination of the care provided for Christine and her family.

Nursing is a process, and one part of the process is no more important that any other part. This process is complex and requires the practitioner to consider both objective and subjective information. Objective facts are gathered from documents and observations. Subjective information is concerned with feelings, emotions, values and beliefs, and this information is obtained from each member of the team, the patient and his or her family. The nursing process should be seen not as a series of steps which are hierarchical or linear, each one following on from the other, but as a spiral – one step linking back to the other. Evaluation needs to be an integral part of each step (usually described as formative evaluation) and an overall reflection when patient care ends or is completed (summative evaluation). You are invited to consider how you would evaluate Christine's care and compare your impressions with those of Rachel.

Nurses' introduction to Christine

Rachel had obtained details about Christine's medical history and her family from Dr Bennett who had been the family's GP for ten years. Dr Bennett worked closely with the primary health care team and during the weekly meeting referred Christine for a nursing assessment and help in dealing with constipation. Rachel decided she would like to try 'adaptation nursing' since she felt the focus on behaviours and the concept of adaptation fitted the community setting. Rachel felt that adaptation was of concern to most of her patients in one way or another.

Christine's parents' house was a neat semi, at the end of a cul-de-sac on the edge of the town. On Rachel's first visit an elderly harassed-looking woman answered the door and without speaking opened it widely to let Rachel in. Without smiling she pointed to the stairs and said 'Christine is still in bed'. She did not follow Rachel upstairs but disappeared down the hall to the end of the house. The house was decorated in a pale neutral way. It had a lived-in appearance but did not seem inviting or homely.

Christine was in bed. Her bedroom was drab but clean, and Rachel was not able to make any assumptions about Christine's personality likes or dislikes from the way her bedroom was furnished and decorated. Rachel sat down on the chair which had been placed beside the bed and introduced herself. Christine was sitting in bed sipping a glass of milk. She had a full round face and huge brown eyes. Her hair was short and she looked much younger than her 36 years. The date of the first visit was the 6th July. What follows is an account of Christine's care during that month of July.

Assessment

Rachel had obtained a detailed description of Christine and her family from Dr Bennett, but she was aware that she needed to understand Christine's perception of the situation. She needed to gather as much information as possible without causing Christine distress physically or emotionally. Rachel decided for the first visit that she would concentrate on Christine's immediate discomfort or problem, which was the constipation. Rachel concentrated on assessing Christine's physiological adaptation on the first visit and continued the assessment of adaptation in the other modes on subsequent visits.

Assessment of behaviours: physiological mode

Oxygenation

Breathing was quiet, regular and without distress; speaking was not a strain and did not cause breathlessness. Christine reported that she became exhausted when walking. At no time did she refer to being breathless but always described the feeling as tired, exhausted, weary or worn out. When she walked to the bathroom, a distance of about 5 metres, Rachel observed how breathless Christine became – her respirations increased from 28 per minute to 80 per minute.

Nutrition

Christine reported that she did not want to eat and was not tempted by any foods. Swallowing was difficult so she did not bother to eat. The last meal she had enjoyed was when she was on holiday four weeks ago. She had felt sick for the last few days but had not vomited. She enjoyed ice cold milk and drank several pints each day. Christine said she had not lost weight and she looked well-rounded. Her skin turgor was satisfactory and she looked tanned and deceptively healthy. She managed to take her tablets by asking her mother to crush them in some milk, which she then drank from a spoon. She said this was satisfactory and she didn't mind the taste.

Fluids and electrolytes

Christine's constipation (one of the main reasons for Dr Bennett's referral) could, if not dealt with, lead to electrolyte imbalance. Adaptation in terms of fluids and electrolytes is described as homeostasis. Rachel knew from experience that the nurse is in an ideal position to detect subtle behavioural changes which might imply an electrolyte imbalance. Any 'suspicions' could then be 'checked out' by a blood test. Christine was hydrated and not vomiting, and because of this Rachel was not over-concerned but she felt the need consciously to monitor any behavioural indications of an imbalance. Changes she looked for were general malaise, restlessness, apathy, irritability, confusion and memory failure. These behaviours are assessed under the heading of neurological function.

Neurological function

Christine was tired but she did not appear agitated or irritable. Rachel thought that, considering her physical discomfort and situation, Christine was calm and pragmatic. During discussions with Christine, Rachel noted that she was able to remember the day of Dr Bennett's last visit and the dates of her operation and treatment.

Activity and rest

Christine could not walk to the bathroom next to her bedroom without becoming breathless. Going downstairs and coming up again was a considerable problem. Her father would usually help her if she wanted to watch television. Rachel noted that Christine did not want, or was unable, to differentiate clearly between breathlessness and tiredness.

Her sister visited every weekend and would wash and dry Christine's hair. Christine and her sister had recently returned from a cruise. The extreme tiredness had started when they returned three weeks ago. The last time she had felt well was on holiday.

Sleeping

This was a problem and Christine found that coughing disturbed her. She also needed to sleep sitting up since the operation, and she felt this was the most comfortable position. Three pillows were piled one on the other against the head of her bed.

Her father had been to the chemist and bought some linctus for the cough. She found the sweetness of the mixture soothing, but it did not seem to help the cough.

Most of the day was spent 'dozing'. Christine often found that she missed the end of radio programmes.

Protection

Christine's skin was intact. She thought it was in good condition because of the sun cream she had been using on holiday. Her pneumonectomy scar had healed with no signs of redness or soreness. There was no residual soreness or redness as a result of the radiotherapy. She had no problems with her teeth as she had always attended the dentist regularly. There was a slight white coating on her tongue possibly owing to the amount of milk that she drank, but her tongue and mouth looked moist. Her hair, although neatly cut, was greasy and lank. Christine found the stretching needed to wash her hair exhausting and she was looking forward to her sister helping her at the weekend.

There were no signs of any infection and base-line temperature pulse and blood pressure were within normal limits at rest.

Senses

Christine answered questions and offered information politely and patiently. She only became expressive when talking about her holiday. During Rachel's visits Christine was always in her bedroom. Occasionally during the evening she would go downstairs to watch television but mostly she said she liked to remain in her room. She liked to listen to her collection of country and western music. She had also become a radio fan and liked to listen to plays and 'chat programmes'. Two weeks ago she had found the Distalgesic she had been taking for the pain in her chest to be ineffective.

Dr Bennett had prescribed morphine sulphate tablets (MST) 12 hourly. Christine thought the new ones were better. She never referred to the tablets by name but used the expression 'the ones for pain or the bowels'. She was afraid of injections and Dr Bennett had assured her that she would not need to have any injections. But she felt worried as she could not take an extra tablet if, for instance, the pain suddenly got worse in the middle of the night.

The pain Christine described as 'in her chest' was over the sternum area. She could not think of a word to describe it and said it was there most of the time. McGaffery's (1979) seminal work describes nursing management for people with pain. McGaffery's definition of pain states 'pain is whatever the experiencing person says it is existing whenever s/he says it is'. This definition illustrates the subjective nature of pain.

Although Rachel accepted Christine's description of 'in her chest and there all the time', she felt the need to help Christine explore her pain. For instance, was there one type of pain, was there an increase in pain on movement? Rachel also needed to help Christine to express the pain in words so that its intensity and duration could be understood. Rachel also understood that patients in chronic pain (pain that is not acute or of short duration) which is not reversible have to combat the depressing factor which exacerbtes the experience of pain.

Assessment of stimuli: physiological mode

Christine's physiological integrity in terms of adaptation was threatened by several factors which can be summarised as follows: constipation, pain, lack of rest and balanced nutrition. Christine's nutritional needs were particularly vitamins and minerals not found in milk. She also needed adequate rest. Rachel was wary of being overwhelmed by considering the assessment of all the stimuli in the physiological mode, so she made the decision to concentrate on one aspect at a time.

Christine had already adapted effectively in a number of ways. She was accepting her fear of 'break through pain'. She had decided not to eat and could not be persuaded to try anything except milk, but needed fruit juice for vitamin C. In dealing with the constipation she was taking the medication regularly, but could not effectively cope with the energy needed to defaecate.

Assessment of behaviour: self-concept mode and physical self

Christine was quiet and unassuming and did not like talking about herself. She described herself as introvert and her sister as extrovert. She did not want to make any demands on anyone, particularly her mother. Christine appeared reluctant to answer any personal questions and rarely during the time Rachel knew her did she volunteer any information. When Christine did talk she would describe how she was feeling physically or about her recent holiday. She became quite animated when showing Rachel the photographs of the holiday and she enjoyed describing the exotic places they had visited.

In terms of development Christine has reached what Erikson (1980) calls the 'grand degenerative function'. For the young person reaching this stage without experiencing old age and gradual degeneration, this means that adaptation needs to be more extreme or active.

Personal self

When answering questions about her likes and dislikes, the information disclosed by Christine was superficial. She was never heard by Rachel to reflect or speculate or wish for anything. Rachel noted that she also changed the subject in order, it seemed, to shift the focus from herself. It seemed inappropriate to ask questions about friends, male or female. Only once during that month did Christine refer to a group of friends visiting her.

All enquiries were dealt with in the present and, apart from showing Rachel pictures of the cruise, Christine did not discuss the past or the future. Rachel felt uneasy about this because she knew from the experience of nursing terminally ill people of all ages that Christine must have considerable anxiety.

Assessment of stimuli: self-concept mode

The assessment began to become difficult for Rachel at this point. She felt that the most important stimulus for Christine was her cancer. Christine would talk about her physical symptoms but it appeared that she had decided not to talk about the past or the future. In response to this chosen way of coping, Rachel felt that she would deal with the 'immediate, here and now'. This was difficult for Rachel because she felt that as a nurse she could help patients anticipate and prevent potential problems. She could of course help Christine deal with physical problems, but she felt excluded from the psychological and emotional ones.

Assessment of behaviour: role function

Roles are usually described as primary, secondary or tertiary. For the purposes of assessment and measuring adaptation, roles need to be seen in terms of behaviours. Christine's primary role was of a young adult: although she was living at home, she made decisions about what she wanted and when.

Before her illness Christine's secondary roles would have been described as daughter, carer for her parents and legal secretary. The only role behaviour Rachel observed was Christine's 'sick role'. When patients adopt a 'sick role' this is often described as a tertiary role, except when the illness is chronic when it becomes a secondary role. If the illness is all-consuming and requires energy and attention to the exclusion of other aspects of life, it can then truly be described as a secondary role.

Although we do not choose to become ill we can choose if we are going to adopt a 'sick role'. The role that Christine seemed to have adopted almost without question was that of the patient.

Roy and Andrews (1991) describe four factors which confirm or act as major stimuli for sick role behaviour. These are: (1) consumer; (2) access to facilities/set of circumstances; (3) co-operation/collaboration; and (4) rewards. Rachel considered the four factors with Christine in mind:

1. *Consumer.* Christine was receiving nursing care from Rachel, medical care from Dr Bennett and attention from her parents. This helped to confirm her role behaviour.
2. *Access to facilities and set of circumstances.* The disease process and becoming ill again, needing and taking medication, were powerful stimuli for 'sick role behaviour' for Christine.
3. *Cooperation/collaboration.* This category refers to the time allowed for the particular role. In terms of time for Christine, it was now an integral part of her life. The amount of time associated with a role acts a stimulus for the behaviour.
4. *Rewards.* Christine had in place a network of care. Her mother and father were also united in a common goal – looking after her. These factors meant the behaviour of a sick person was reinforced and rewarded.

The 'sick role' was first described by Parsons (1966) and has become a generally accepted term for nurses. Rachel reflected on how uncomfortable she felt in assessing this aspect of Christine's life and analysing it. It felt as if she was applying a stereotypical label, Rachel had always endeavoured to avoid describing people using labels, as she felt it detracted from individuality or the person being a 'universe of one' (Erikson, 1963).

In response to the query about the past, Christine would reply 'I couldn't manage it now, just going next door exhausts me'. It appeared that Christine was able to manage herself in the present without reference to the past or the future. The role that she was immersed in seemed absorbing and she seemed to be coping in a resigned and pragmatic way.

Assessment of stimuli: role mastery

Christine's illness and her physical symptoms were the main stimuli in this mode. As we have discussed, the sick role had become a secondary role. Rachel speculated that there seemed to be a good case for proposing that the sick role had almost become Christine's primary role. Christine's parents taking on the caring role was also an important stimulus. Christine before her illness had 'cared' for her father, and her mother was the sick person. Roles were now reversed. Christine did not seem to have any role conflict.

Assessment of behaviour: interdependence

Christine gave very few clues as to how she felt about the other people in her life. She talked about looking forward to her sister's visits at the weekend and how good it was to have her mother home.

She asked her mother for all the things she needed and did not seem to mind asking for what she wanted despite having said that she did not want to be a bother to her mother. Her mother attended to all of Christine's requests for drinks, crushing up the medication and attending to these requests with quiet obedience, but did not make any suggestions or have any notion about anticipating needs.

Christine accepted help and suggestions from Rachel in a quiet, resigned and dignified way. Rachel thought Christine's behaviour was accepting and fatalistic, yet she did not appear powerless. Rachel's perception of her and her situation was that Christine had given up, but in a strange way she seemed to be in control. She often asked to be left alone and she then retreated into herself. At no time did she become sullen or angry or display any 'negative' feelings, but equally she did not appear to be unbearably angelic. Although she seemed alone, paradoxically she did not appear lonely and isolated. She did not appear to resent being dependent on her parents or Rachel.

Assessment of stimuli: interdependence mode

Christine's dependence seemed to be a necessity. She needed her parents, her sisters and Rachel's help. She also seemed to expect and accept her parent's care and assistance. Rachel wondered if Christine's parents felt a sense of satisfaction and achievement in caring for their child again.

Nursing diagnosis

Roy and Andrews (1991) define nursing diagnosis as 'a judgement process resulting in a statement conveying the person's adaptation process'. It involves stating the behaviour and the most relevant stimuli. Rachel was not used to using nursing diagnosis and was concerned about the care planning not being extensive enough. Although on reflection she did seem to have all relevant information.

The second concern for Rachel was the absence of a nursing diagnosis that addressed the self-concept, role mastery and inter-dependent modes. Rachel felt that Christine's had adapted effectively in these modes but had 'nagging' anxieties about having missed something. Rachel would like to have changed some of the environmental stimuli to make Christine's surroundings more attractive and stimulating, but she was powerless to change any of these aspects of Christine's life. It may have been possible if Mr or Mrs Jacobs had stopped to speak to her – she might then have made some suggestions. They appeared to see Rachel as Christine's nurse and seemed reluctant to approach her. Rachel knew Dr Bennett talked to them when she visited.

Goal setting

Goal statements may be described as measurement of behaviours which confirm adaptation. Rachel did not find identifying the goals in terms of behaviour to be a problem. Although she did not set goals concerning self-concept, she was beginning to think about how changes in self-concept role and interdependence could be expressed in terms of behaviours (see Table 5.1 for details of the care plan). Community nursing, unlike hospital nursing, relies on the patient and the relatives to achieve the goals. Rachel felt that goals which clearly state behaviour helped patients to understand more easily the changes expected and to aim for. Christine agreed with Rachel's ideas for the goals identified.

Table 5.1 *Christine's care plan using Roy's six step nursing process (adapted from Riehl and Roy, 1980)*

Assessment behaviour	Assessment stimuli (F – Local; C – Contextual; R – Residual)	Nursing diagnosis	Goal statement	Intervention	Date and evaluation
Breathless and exhausted when walking a few metres Constipated and unable to defaecate due to exhaustion	F. Christine has cancer C. Feels uncomfortable and nauseous R. Electrolyte imbalance	Christine is constipated and cannot defaecate due to breathlessness	Christine will have bowel action every 3 days	• Phosphate enema every 3 days • Allow 45 min. • Christine will walk to bathroom • Christine will use relaxation and breathing exercises • Christine will walk back and rest • Foot massage to help Christine to relax	10th July No discomfort or sickness 20th July Regime satisfactory, no sickness
Difficulty in swallowing and has decided not to eat	F. Cannot swallow solid food C. Only drinks milk because she is afraid of vomiting R. Thrush and mouth ulcers	Christine needs to drink fruit juice and maintain her fluid intake at 1.5 litres a day	Christine will drink 25 ml of fruit juice and water after milk drinks to cleanse her mouth	• Inform reasons for fluid intake • Identify number of glasses of fluid each day • Monitor amount and colour of urine (Christine will do this) • Ask Christine to repeat reasons for drinking fruit juice and water • Ask Christine to state reasons for maintaining fluid intake	12th July Christine has fruit juice on most days 15th July Christine realises that fluids may prevent sickness 20th July Tongue only slightly coated but mouth moist
Can only walk a few metres Pain in chest – there most the time	F. Sleep disrupted by pain and coughing C. Worried about 'break through pain'	Christine is exhausted and needs to rest	Christine will identify factors which prevent her from sleeping for 3 hours at a time	• Keep a symptom chart • Explain about sleeping for 2–3 hours a time for rest • Ask Dr B for elixir	10th July Christine too tired to complete chart. Discuss each day

84

Table 5.1 continued

Assessment behaviour	Assessment stimuli (F – Local; C – Contextual; R – Residual)	Nursing diagnosis	Goal statement	Intervention	Date and evaluation
Sleep disrupted by coughing	R. Pain is irreversible and chronic			• Continue to take linctus • Complete symptom chart • Use eucalyptus oil and burner at night 10th July Discuss previous days' symptoms and amount of medication 23rd July Christine will take 5 ml of elixir if coughing at night	20th July Noticed coughing and worry associated. Will try relaxation exercises 23rd July Relaxation not working Dr Bennett suggests 5 ml of elixir at night if coughing 25th July Now has several hours' undisturbed sleep at night and during the day

Implementation

The 'bathroom regime' worked well. Following a brief discussion with Christine about what action could be taken, it was decided to use a small phosphate enema. Christine thought she would find waiting for suppositories to work 'excruciating'. Rachel decided to use an enema every three days because she did not consider that in the short term, at least, Christine's energy or breathlessness would improve. Christine and Rachel established a partnership for the 'bathroom sessions', since Christine refused the use of a commode. Christine would walk to the bathroom and then rest for a while. Rachel would then administer the enema and stay with Christine, helping her to relax by getting her to concentrate on her breathing. Christine was afraid to be alone as she felt she would not be able to cope. With practice the relaxation and breathing improved, and this meant that Christine had enough 'energy' to walk back to her room. Rachel found that a way of helping Christine to relax on return to her bedroom was to give her a foot massage using some hand cream. This worked well and Rachel would often leave Christine asleep. Uncharacteristically, one day Christine added 'I find you a great comfort' to her usual 'thank you'.

Although Christine needed help from Rachel with the enema, this regime worked and she did not report any further abdominal discomfort or nausea. Rachel felt the partnership aspect of the regime involved alteration of the stimuli, i.e. not being able to expel the faeces, the adaptation Christine achieved was by relaxing and breathing exercises.

The other stimuli that Rachel needed to consider was Christine's pain, the cough and her nutritional needs. Rachel was uncertain how to continue as she felt she needed to have more explicit information. Rachel could see that behaviours in one mode affected the other modes. Several factors were influencing Christine's need for rest and, in order to help adapt effectively to her exhaustion, she agreed to ask Dr Bennett to prescribe morphine elixir for 'break through pain'. She could also record on the 'symptom chart' when she had 'break through pain' as well as the word which described the pain.

Christine would also record what she was doing when she started to cough. She decided to continue with the linctus and to use eucalyptus oil in an essential oil burner that her sister had bought but which had never been used.

She considered whether the coughing could be associated with any particular activity such as drinking or anxiety. Perhaps Christine's glands in her chest were inflamed, in which case Dr Bennett could be asked to prescribe some steroids. Christine did manage to make an association between the coughing and anxiety. Unfortunately, relaxation did not help and Christine followed Dr Bennett's suggestion of taking a spoonful of mixture.

Christine's fear of 'break through pain' and having no medication to deal with it was satisfied by having Dr Bennett prescribe an elixir for emergency use.

Rachel wanted to ask Christine to keep a 'symptom diary' but felt she would not have the energy to write out what she was experiencing. So it was decided that Rachel would make out a chart and Christine would tick against a time column when she had pain and what word best described it. Rachel and Christine compiled a list of commonly used words to describe pain. She also compiled a list of words so that Christine could be aware of when and what she was doing when she began coughing (see Table 5.2 for details of the symptom chart). This chart was not entirely successful as Christine did not have the energy to complete it. Rachel used it to review the previous day's symptoms and found it useful in discussing Christine's symptoms.

Table 5.2 *Symptom chart*

Time	Medication	Pain level	Pain code	Cough	Code	(Words and levels decided by Christine)
						MEDICATION: T = MST E = Elixir L = Linctus PAIN LEVEL: 1. No pain 2. Some pain 3. Severe pain 4. Awful pain 5. As much as I can bear PAIN WORDS: 6. Sharp 7. Nagging 8. Grinding 9. Throbbing 10. Stabbing 11. Burning 12. Aching 13. Gnawing COUGHING ASSOCIATED WITH: a. Worrying b. Washing/Dressing c. Walking d. Drinking e. Talking f. Medicine

Towards the end of July, Rachel was due to go on holiday. She discussed this with Dr Bennett who thought this would be a good opportunity for Christine to have a few weeks' respite care. She also thought that Mr and Mrs Jacobs needed a rest. A GP bed was booked for Christine in the local hospital. Christine with her usual stoicism accepted the idea.

Rachel was pleased to have helped Christine to establish increased adaptation patterns of behaviour and therefore increased control. A visit to the ward of the hospital and a discussion with the sister confirmed that they would use Christine's care plan and she could continue to take her own medication.

On the 31st of July Christine was admitted to the ward. Her sister had made a special journey to wash her hair and her father drove her to the hospital. Rachel visited Christine that evening to say goodbye and took her some flowers from her garden. Rachel smiled as she walked into the ward. Christine was sitting up in bed drinking a glass of milk. She looked comfortable and said she liked the bright four-bedded ward and could see out of the windows. Rachel said goodbye and assured her of a visit after her holiday.

When Rachel returned from holiday, Dr Bennett informed her that Christine had died at 4 am on the 1st August.

Evaluation

Rachel felt hurt and disappointed that Christine had died while she was on holiday. She realised that she must set aside this rather selfish personal view in order to evaluate Christine's care and death from a nursing perspective.

Evaluation is more than considering whether the goals are achieved. Roy and Andrews (1991) define evaluation as 'judging the effectiveness of nursing intervention in relation to the person's behaviour.' Rachel had recently become convinced that she must learn as much as she could from her experience in order to improve her knowledge and skills.

Roy and Andrews (1991) believe that people are both creative and purposeful. It was this idea of all people organising and managing their existence in the best way they could that first attracted Rachel to Roy's model. Rachel had noticed that even when patients were not obviously managing their problems but denying or ignoring whatever was confronting them, they still in different ways adapted to cope with their situation. Even ignoring the problem is a way of coping with it.

Roy and Andrews (1991) consider that behaviour is deliberate – people are not seen as just haphazardly reacting to their lives. The overall goal of adaptation nursing is the integrity of the patient. Rachel felt that this·meant a balance between the stimulus on the one hand and the person's ability to cope effectively on the other. The nursing role is to encourage integrity by either changing the stimulus or helping the person to change to more effective coping behaviours. Rachel felt the way to judge the effectiveness of Christine's behaviour in relation to the nursing intervention was to assess whether Christine's behaviour indicated a degree of integrity in each of Roy's four modes.

Considering the *physiological mode*, Rachel thought that the enema changed the stimuli. Christine's behaviour had changed because she did not feel sick and uncomfortable, and by maintaining her fluid balance integrity in terms of homeostasis was achieved. She was also able to conserve some energy by using the relaxation exercises. Christine's need for rest was more difficult to satisfy and she did not achieve two or three hours' sound sleep until she made an association between the coughing and her anxiety.

Several hours' uninterrupted sleep is important if it is to be restorative and protective (Hodgson, 1991). The symptom chart had been a good idea, as it had been a useful tool in discussing Christine's pain, coughing and anxiety. Rachel knew from experience that patients often found describing their feelings difficult. She realised that it was a hard task for most people to find the words to describe inner and deeply personal and private experiences.

As regards the *self-concept*, Christine's only mention of anxiety was to say she sometimes felt afraid and then she changed the subject. Remembering this made Rachel reflect on how she had responded and if she could have facilitated an exploration of Christine's fears. Rachel did feel she could have been more open about discussing these fears. There may have been the anticipation of greater pain or the process or act of dying. Rachel wondered if some nurses might have seen Christine's reticence as 'not coping effectively', and that Rachel should have been more insistent in talking about the future. Dr Bennett also felt she had provided Christine with an opportunity to talk about her fears, but Christine had not indicated that she wished to talk.

Christine's symptom chart revealed that she had only had to take the elixir twice at night to relieve the coughing. It was at night when Christine had felt afraid. Rachel thought that making the association and understanding why she was coughing helped her to cope with it. Rachel felt when thinking about Christine and the self-concept mode that she had not gained any information about how Christine saw herself apart from her saying she was an introvert.

Roy's concept of *role mastery* helped Rachel to deepen her understanding of the sick role. She had always felt that it was a negative character trait and a poor coping strategy. Rachel had to admit to wishing Christine would be more independent and to have more 'fight', but the reality was that she achieved the level of independence possible for her, so she accepted the only role available to her with dignity.

The *interdependence mode* of Roy's model has evolved and now has a different focus. McIntier (1976) described interdependence as 'the comfortable balance between dependence and independence in relationship with others.' This was how Rachel had understood and used the idea of interdependence. The problem with this view was that Rachel found that she often polarised the two types of behaviour, the dependent and the independent. A judgement then needed to be made about the balance. Roy and Andrews (1991) acknowledge clarification and developments by other nurse theorists and now define interdependence as 'the close relationship of people that involves the willingness to love, respect and value others and to respond to love, respect and value given by others.' Randell *et al.* (1982) believe that during infancy two adaptive modes are important – the physiological and the interdependence mode. They observed elderly people admitted to centres in their final years. This group of people were found to give up their previously held roles and ideas of themselves, through self-concept.

The authors suggest that the physiological and interdependence modes are the first to be acquired during infancy and are given up last. Reading about this helped Rachel to appreciate many aspects of Christine's care; she gave and received respect, value and love. She accepted the developmental task of dying with quiet resolve but without discussing it. Rachel described this as fatalistic. Fatalism is described as a coping strategy by Moorey and Greer (1989), and is not thought to be maladaptive but rather one way of dealing with a situation. Christine's energy was transferred from living for a future life to dealing with the present (Leick and Davidsen-Nielsen, 1991). In terms of adaptation this was positive. Christine had so little energy emotionally or physically that she needed instinctively to be as economical as she could with what she had.

Overall Rachel felt she had helped Christine to achieve certain levels of adaptation. Christine's adaptation had been thought out to accord with what Roy and Andrews (1991) call cognator adaptation. Regulator adaptation was the pain, tiredness and breathlessness which made Christine conserve her energy. The way Rachel had helped was in terms of helping Christine make associations, i.e. the coughing, and to cope with constipation and the pain. She felt she had helped to prevent complications such as endocrine imbalance and mouth problems such as thrush. Rachel was aware of knowing little about what Christine thought – her psychological 'black box' remained private and Rachel did not know to what extent her adaptation to death was about how she thought about it. Rachel wondered why she died in hospital? Was it because hospitals are places where people die? Did Christine need privacy away from her parents and Rachel in order to die?

Rachel was still left with the question: could she have been more effective? One thing she felt that she could have changed was her response to Mr and Mrs Jacobs. With hindsight, Rachel felt that she avoided them. They regarded her as Christine's nurse and she was happy to leave it like that. Thinking about them later she acknowledged that she felt a little worried by Mrs Jacob's psychiatric history (another label). She did regret not having established some form of relationship with them, but she had reconciled this to herself at the time by thinking that Dr Bennett knew them and could keep them informed and answer their questions. Rachel felt that using Roy's model had provided her with a 'macro and a micro view' of Christine. The 'macro' or whole view was aided by assessing behaviours and stimuli in all four modes. Each mode affects the others and, in order to view coping strategies, the modes can be seen as interrelated. This dovetailing of the separate modes makes a comprehensive whole. However, a 'microscopic' or narrow view is useful in order to focus on the types of stimuli. Care can then be targeted accurately to aid effective adjustment or adaptation.

Questions

1. Rachel was upset at not being able to say goodbye to Christine before she died, and this raises significant issues about the purpose of nursing and what makes for satisfying practice. If you were in Rachel's situation, how would you deal with this disappointment?

2. The notion of 'adaptation' during the process of dying can seem

strange. After all, finally the patient's capacity to adapt is finite. Nevertheless, there are aspects of adaptation present, drawing upon cognator and regulator functions. Can you offer examples from each, using Christine's story?

3. Rachel was unsure of her success in relating to Christine's parents. They after all provided a great deal of support and fulfilled role functions that Rachel could not attend to, given her formal nursing commitments. To what extent do you think Rachel could have negotiated a different role toward Christine's parents? (You might wish to list the stressors that limited Rachel's role function.)

4. Interdependence is about giving and receiving – developing the skills and grace to share in life imaginatively and with trust. Christine faced the challenge of becoming a care receiver – her mother a care deliverer. To what extent do you think Christine's age and single status, and her mother's illness, affected this new set of interdependent roles?

5. Roy assumes that people are creative, and their behaviour is purposeful. What evidence exists in this study to illustrate creative thought in action?

Learning/teaching activities and exercises

1. This study has been all about loss and dignity – the nurse's role in assisting Christine to choose adaptive responses to her deteriorating health. It suggests the question: what is a 'quality death' and what part does nursing care, professional care, play within that?

   In discussion with colleagues, devise a list of 10 characteristics that highlight what a 'quality death' might mean. For instance, you might emphasise the fullest respect for the patient's preferences in matters of toilet and hygiene. Then discuss the following two questions collectively.

   (a) To what extent does my view on this result from:
      • nurse education
      • my personal socialisation, at home and in school
      • my cultural and religious perspective?
      (You will be mapping some of the residual stimuli that set the scene as you deliver palliative care!)

   (b) How easy was it to arrive at a list of 10 characteristics? In short, is it easy to define a good death? (If not, perhaps you might wonder why!)

This exercise should take approximately 90 minutes. It is recommended to take 45 minutes to draw up the list of 10 characteristics, and a further 45 minutes to discuss responses to the two questions. Use a comfortable environment, with refreshments and easy chairs to facilitate this important discussion.

The next activity can be done individually or as a group. It concerns loss, and you are asked to complete the exercise and then consider how you would adapt to loss. You may also like to think about how the loss may affect other parts of your life. Although this exercise may be uncomfortable it provides a useful opportunity to think about the implications of loss and adaptation to it.

2. This exercise can be undertaken in a group or individually. It involves dealing with loss – anybody who is currently immersed in a personal loss situation is advised not to participate. How to use the exercise as an individual will be described first.

Equipment: Each person will need:

- nine small pieces of paper
- a pen or pencil
- a large pad or A4 paper to record responses

Step 1

(a) On one side of each piece of paper, write your name:

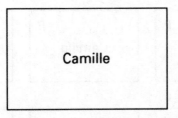

(b) Add on the same side as your name the following:
    (i) on three pieces, in the right-hand corner add the letter B
    (ii) on another three, add the letter P
    (iii) and finally on the last three, add the letter S.

Step 2

On the reverse side of the papers marked B, identify and write

93

down three aspects of your biological/physical self that you value – write one on each sheet of paper. These values may be simple like movement or walking, or complex like dancing or playing squash.

Step 3
On the reverse side of the pieces of paper marked P, identify and write down three aspects of your psychological self that you value, one on each piece of paper. This part of the self is concerned with emotions: thinking, motivation and character traits – for example 'happy'.

Step 4
Lastly, on the reverse side of the papers marked S, identify and write down values concerned with the social self. These aspects include titles, roles, status, social activities, pastimes and hobbies – for example 'married'.

Step 5
When all nine items have been identified, place them in groups with the name and identifying letters uppermost:

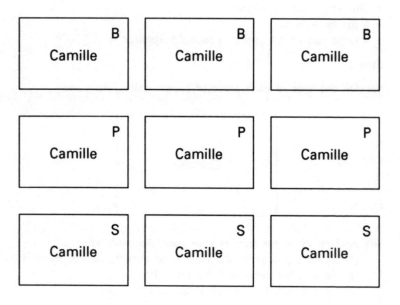

Step 6
Remove one card from each group and put them to one side. Turn over the removed cards one at a time, starting with B.

Step 7
First consider the biological. What aspect of your biological self has been removed and therefore lost? What would your life be like without this part of yourself? Write this down.

What are the first things that come into your mind? Write them down.

Perhaps adaptation in the short term would be difficult or impossible.
How might you be helped to adapt to living life without this? What stages or planning might be required?

What would your world be like without these values?

How would you adapt to the loss?

Step 8
Think through the implication carefully and write your comments and thoughts. Writing down and reading them back will help the thought process.

Work through steps 6 and 7 for the psychological self and the social self. Answer the same questions for the losses of these values.

Step 9
Consider how patients who experience similar losses cope with their feelings.

How do patients cope with strong feelings?

Are the patient's feelings ever acknowledged?

Is the validity of having these strong feelings ever accepted?

When you have completed your individual reflections, pick up the pieces of paper that identify the losses, along with the others.

How does it feel to be whole again?

What is it like to have the values all together?

When you have completed this exercise, consider what are you going to do with the pieces of paper with your values written on them.

Using this values exercise with a group or in pairs:
Explain that this exercise is about dealing with loss and that if anyone wants to leave and not take part, they may.
This needs to be done in an open way, so that anyone who wishes to leave does not feel guilty.
Equipment as before.
Give instructions for step 1.
Relate steps 2, 3 and 4 to the group, allowing time for people to make decisions about what they would like to identify.
Complete step 5.
Explain to the group that their cards will not be looked at or read out.
Once all the cards or pieces of paper are set out, remove one card from each group B, P and S, and set them to one side.
Ask the group to think firstly about what they have lost in the biological group. Answer questions in step 7 and complete step 8. Then complete steps 7 and 8 for the psychological self and the social self.
Discuss in pairs the answers to the questions in step 7. How do you feel about the exercise?
Ask the group now to identify how they feel about you, the teacher. You have removed their values and have them. What might you do with them?
A flip-chart may be used to list the feelings expressed by the members of the group:

- anger
- fear
- frustration
- helplessness etc.

Discuss with the group how patients cope with their strong feelings about loss. Are their feelings acknowledged, or accepted?
Give back the values without looking at them. Discuss with the group how it feels to have their values back – to be whole again.
Decide as a group what to do with the pieces of paper.

A group may finish with each member considering and completing the sentence 'At the end of this exercise I have learnt . . .'

REFERENCES

For Roy's Model – a basis for a helping relationship

Benner, P. and Wrubel, J. (1989) *The Primacy of Caring.* Menlo Park, California: Addison-Wesley.

Cawley, S. (1991) A symbolic awareness context identified through a grounded theory study of health visiting. *Journal of Advanced Nursing*, **16**, 148–656.

Foster, M. and Mayall, B. (1990) Health visitors as educators, *Journal of Advanced Nursing*, **15**, 286–292.

Henwood, M. (1987) The family and the home, an occasional paper, pp 9–18. London: Family Policy Studies Centre.

Morse, J. (1992) Beyond empathy: expanding expressions of caring. *Journal of Advanced Nursing*, **17**, 809–821.

Price, B. (1987) First impressions paradigms for patient assessment. *Journal of Advanced Nursing*, **12**, 699–705.

Roy, C. and Andrews, H. (1991) *The Roy Adaptation Model, the Definitive Statement.* Norwalk, Connecticut: Appleton & Lange.

Royal College of Midwives (1991) *Successful Breast Feeding*, 2nd edn. Edinburgh: Churchill Livingstone.

Thompson, D. (1990) Too busy for assessments. *Nursing*, **4**(21), 35.

Tierney, A. (1984) *Open University 553: A Systematic Approach to Nursing Care.* Milton Keynes: Open University Press.

Winnicot, D. (1986) *Home Is Where We Start From.* Harmondsworth, Middlesex: Penguin.

For Christine – a study in interdependence

Erikson, E. (1963) *Childhood and Society.* New York: Norton.

Erikson, E. (1980) *Identity and the Life Cycle.* New York: Norton.

Hodgson, L. (1991) Why do we need sleep? Relating theory to practice. *Journal of Advanced Nursing*, **16**, 1503–1510.

Leick, N. and Davidsen-Nielsen, M. (1991) *Healing Pain*, p 163. London: Routledge.

McGaffery, M. (1979) *Nursing Management of Patients with Pain.* Philadelphia, Pennsylvania: Lippincott.

McIntier, T. (1976) Theory of interdependence. Cited in Fawcett, J., *Analysis of Conceptual Models of Nursing.* Philadelphia, Pennsylvania: Davis, 1984.

Moorey, S. and Greer, S. (1989) *Psychological Therapy from Patients with Cancer*, p 10. Oxford: Heinemann.

Parsons, T. (1966) On becoming a patient. In Folker, K. and Deck, E. (Eds), *A Sociological Framework for Patient Care*. New York: Wiley.

Randell, B., Tedrow, M. and Van Landingham, J. (1982) *Adaptation Nursing, the Roy Conceptual Model Applied*. St Louis, Missouri: Mosby.

Riehl, J. and Roy, C. (1980) *Conceptual Models for Nursing Practice*, 2nd edn. Norwalk, Connecticut: Appleton-Century Croft.

Roy, C. and Andrews, H. (1991) *The Roy Adaptation Model, the Definitive Statement*. Norwalk, Connecticut: Appleton & Lange.

CHAPTER SIX

Applying the Model III
Greg Cox

SURGERY WITH STOMA FORMATION

'The problem started only six weeks ago. I had mucousy blood in my faeces, not painful. I thought this is not right, so I went to my GP who sent me to see the Hospital Consultant. He examined me. I went back to him a week later. Well, John, he said, you will need an operation that will mean a bag. I knew what he meant, I felt disgusted. I replied 'No, I don't want that'. I remember he paused and then said 'Well John, it's either a bag or a coffin'. That shook me. I thought of my wife, we've been married for 60 years. I thought, better a bag and a few more years with her. There's no choice'.

During this interview, behaviours such as John sighing, holding his head down and at times avoiding eye contact were noted. He also mentioned, in passing, a fear of not getting home and how he would cope after the surgery. 'I am 80 years old you know'.

John and Florence live in a bungalow he bought after retiring as a carpenter. He leads, as he describes, a simple but contented life. His neighbours are close friends and he has a small but close-knit social group.

He does have children, but they moved away from the UK with their families some years ago. Florence is also 80 years old – she looks frail but is able to look after herself. However, she would not be able to look after John physically, if this need were to occur.

This study attempts to explore and highlight the nursing care given from John's admission to hospital to his discharge home. An emphasis towards the care given to his psychological needs has been adopted. However, this should not indicate that his physical needs take less of a priority. Staff Nurse James, the primary nurse for

John Goodman, took on the responsibility for the management and guidance of care throughout his stay on an Acute Surgical Ward.

Because of John's situation, his proposed major surgical intervention and his altered body image, the nursing staff considered Roy's Model appropriate. Indeed, Blackmore (1988) suggests that to contribute to the positive adaptation of altered body image, nurses must explore ways of assessing whether positive or negative adaptation has taken place and to identify each patient's coping mechanisms. One way of doing this is to use a nursing model which has a self-concept component, such as Roy's Model. In addition, the comprehensive use of knowledge from other disciplines treating the person 'holistically', affecting the bio-psycho-social being, seemed wholly appropriate and suited John's needs.

In John's case, he was a totally independent 80 year old man, undergoing an unexpected period of dependence upon nursing care for 2–5 days post-operatively, with a gradual return to independence during convalescence. Many factors would be affecting his recovery, and he would have a diversity of stresses and adaptations to contend with.

Admission

Two days before the operation date, John arrived on the ward. He carried a small battered suitcase, and was closely followed by his frail looking wife, Florence. He looked slightly lost and timid. Staff Nurse James had previously arranged with the other members of staff that John would be under his nursing care, and he was therefore expecting him. The couple were shown to a side room with an adjoining toilet, which had been set aside for John's stay. Staff Nurse James realised that for John and Florence this was an anxious time. To help reduce this feeling of insecurity and unfamiliarity, produced by being admitted into a hospital environment, certain steps were taken. These included allowing John and Florence time to settle, introducing those staff participating in his care, giving both John and his wife the opportunity to talk about his anxieties and fears in a calm, relaxed and, if necessary, private environment and, perhaps most important of all, being receptive to their anxiety. In addition, this would help to lay a firm foundation to a good working relationship.

During the initial interview with John and his wife, much two-way communication took place. It was a chance for John to get to know Staff Nurse James and vice versa, ask preliminary questions and also to initiate Roy's first-level assessment. The purpose of this assessment was discussed and explained to John. The interview took an informal approach, with the gathering of information in a relaxed spontaneous manner. However, some direct questions were asked to clarify specific details. During this phase of admission, many personal and sensitive topics about John were to be discussed, and a sensitive approach was needed to ensure the meaningful and positive progression of care to take place. This particularly applies when dealing with the psychological and social aspects, such as his feelings about himself, his body image, and his relationship with Florence. His admission two days prior to his operation gave the opportunity for time to be spent in forming a relationship, gathering information and initiating care.

Roy's first level of assessment

This is the first step in the nursing process and is of vital importance, for without effective assessment, that is, the gaining of necessary information, individualised and effective nursing care would be inhibited.

The goal of nursing, according to Roy, is to promote John's adaptation to the stressors that are and will confront him, that is coming into hospital, cancer, impending surgery, pain and so on. Staff Nurse James needed to determine the extent to which John was able to meet the demands put upon him in order to assist towards his positive adaptation, and thus his coming to terms with them. In assessing John's behaviours, i.e. his responses to stressors, Staff Nurse James used as a format the four adaptive modes as described by Roy.

From the statements and observations made of John's behaviours, i.e. verbal and non-verbal cues such as words, tone of voice and body posture, the following tentative statements were made:

Self-concept mode (how John feels about himself)

- John shows signs of resignation over impending stoma formation.
- By the time of the interview, John had become more resigned for 'what was best for him' although he seemed to show an apathetic attitude.
- John was expressing feelings of powerlessness (lack of control), i.e. with statements such as 'why me?' and 'there's no choice' and 'I have always been a fit man'.

- He was also expressing feelings of disgust at the prospect of a stoma.
- John had mentioned he had known a couple of people who had similar operations approximately 20 years ago and expressed worry about the odour from a stoma.
- John had indicated there was no pain involved at present, but his change of bowel habit was obviously causing upset.
- He expressed concern about the outcome from surgery.
- John has feelings of worry about being in hospital, saying he has never been in one before.

Concerns

- Impending stoma formation.
- Showing signs of incomplete grieving.
- John's concern over his state of health.
- John's concern over ability to cope with stoma.
- John's fear of ability to cope with surgery.
- Insufficient knowledge at present to understand capability to cope with stoma.
- Potential ineffective response to impending change in body image, related to colostomy formation.

Role function mode

Primary	Male, 80 years
	Mature adult
Secondary	Husband – close relationship
	Grandfather, but has no social contact with grandchildren
	Friends, with neighbours, small social group
	Parent – no social contact with children
Tertiary	Gardener, retired carpenter

John expresses concern he will not be the same husband after the operation. The sexual aspect has no concern. There is more concern over being a burden to his wife.

John seems to play a dominant role in the partnership, i.e. being the supportive husband to Florence. He now fears having to be the supported one in their relationship.

John expresses feelings of concern and anxiety about how Florence will cope during his hospital stay. They have not been separated from each other for many years. Whilst in hospital he will not be able to fulfil his husband role. He is unsure of what is expected of him.

Interdependence mode

- John has sought medical care from his doctor, i.e. GP and Consultant. He has agreed to hospitalisation and consequent treatment.
- John's neighbours are close friends.
- He has been married for 60 years.
- His pension is his main income, although he seems to manage on this.
- He has his own bungalow.
- He continues to have a keen interest in gardening.
- There seems to be no other persons or support systems except for neighbours.
- John is unsure how the operation will affect his independence: 'Will I be able to manage?'
- He is an independent person.
- At present John is co-operating with nurses and doctors in his care and he seems pleased to do so.

Role/interdependence

Strengths and concerns – summary

Strengths	A strong bond between John and Florence
	A strong will to return home
	Seeking and accepting need for surgery
Concerns	John's concern for Florence at home
	Convalescence period after discharge from hospital
	Insufficient knowledge at present to understand events concerning surgery
	Temporary loss of independence related to hospital admission

Physiological mode

As well as the psycho-social aspect, i.e. the self-concept, role function and interdependence modes, John was going to have many

103

physical stressors put upon him. The intended major surgery, the anaesthesia, as well as the post-operative recovery period would certainly be causing many stresses which would challenge John's physical adaptive processes. A comprehensive assessment was taken to ensure that possible eventualities could be catered for.

Oxygenation

First-level assessment

John is awake, and alert. He is orientated to reality, i.e. time, persons and place.

> BP 160/90   Pulse 80   Respiration 20
> Pulse regular and full. Respirations are rhythmic and easy, with no effort.
> Normal chest movement

No complaints of shortness of breath. Clear unobstructive airway – no wheeze. Non-smoker – gave up 30 years ago – no medical reason.

Concerns

For anaesthetic in two days. Breathing may be restricted post-operatively, as a result of pain and anaesthetics. 80 years old – age must be considered.

Elimination

First-level assessment

Urine – voids about 4–5 times daily. Total amount: about 1500 ml.

> Normal characteristics: pH 6   Sg 1010
> No glucose, no protein.
> Continent. Can stop and start urine stream. Voids easily. No pain or discomfort.

Dry skin, with no visible perspiration. Temperature 36.8°C.
Bowel – has had irregular bowel habit for previous 6–7 weeks.
4–6 times daily, passing mucous, blood stool. Has control but needs to rush at times. No pain.

Concerns

Cancer of bowel (colon).

Impending surgery, catheterisation post-surgery. Colostomy management post-surgery.

Nutrition

First-level assessment

Height: 5'8"
Weight: 71.3 kg – within normal limits

Expresses no appreciable weight loss. Not obese. Abdomen flat. No special diets. Describes a well-balanced diet.

Skin has texture of 80 year old. Skeleton looks well formed. Wears false teeth. Expresses no problems with eating. Blood glucose 4.5 mmols.

Concerns

No problems at present. Adaptive.
Impending abdominal bowel surgery with consequent nil by mouth for period of days.
No experience of colostomy management concerning diet.

Activity and rest

First-level assessment

No disfigurement of body. Good muscle size for age. Generally smooth co-ordinated movement, deliberate and purposeful. Hand movements – has difficulty in fine sensitive movements. No undue restriction of body movements.

Carries out activities of daily living, i.e. dresses himself, feeds himself, washes himself, grooms himself, controls elimination function (although altered). Mobilises without assistance, i.e. steady, has normal gait.

Rest

Sleeps normally 6–7 hours. Less at present, 4–5 hours. Asleep by 11.00 pm, awake 6.00 am. Wakes during the night 1–2 times. No sedatives used. Does not normally nap during day.

Concerns

Upcoming, i.e. co-ordination of fine movements. Management of colostomy.

Fluids and electrolytes

First-level assessment

Daily intake: 1.5–2 litres
Urine normal: i.e. colour straw and consistency
No unusual retention of fluid, i.e. oedema of feet, ankles, eyelids, sacrum, ascites.

Skin: warm and dry. Maintains normal weight.

Urea and electrolyte laboratory values are:

Sodium	138	mEq/l
Potassium	4.1	mEq/l
Calcium	102	mEq/l
Chloride	102	mEq/l

Pink moist mucous membranes. No apparent impairment of muscles or brain function.

Concerns

Surgery and period of nil by mouth in two days.
   Will need bowel preparation which includes:

1. Low residue diet commencing 2 days post-operatively, then clear fluids only one day prior.
2. Mannatol 20%, 200 ml orally prescribed by physician.

Sensory regulation

First-level assessment

Vision – good sight – does wear glasses, sees well with them.
No other observable defects.
Hearing – hears voices within normal range.
Speech formation and perception – speaks clearly, initiates and understands language.
Sense of touch – slight difficulty in delicate movements.
At ease, comfortable. No pain. Temperature normal, 36.8°C.
Intact healthy skin. Has texture and elasticity of 80 year old.
Endocrine regulation – no apparent abnormalities.

Concerns

Potential infection. Surgical incision, catheterisation.
Chest infection.
Sensory: pain post-operatively.

Second-level assessment

The first-level assessment highlighted John's behaviours that were adaptive or maladaptive (promoting a well-being or distracting from it). Staff Nurse James set about assessing the factors that might directly or indirectly have an influence on these behaviours.

This second-level assessment involves identifying the focal, contextual and residual stimuli which would be affecting the presenting behaviour. As can be seen (Tables 6.1 to 6.4) these are not confined to one adaptive mode, which can influence John in many ways, because of their interlinking nature. These identified stimuli will be the focus of attention for Staff Nurse James.

Table 6.1 *Second-level assessment – John Goodman (Part 1)*

Behaviour	Focal	Contextual	Residual
Feelings of anxiety as shown by:	Hospitalisation	Inadequate knowledge	80 years old
	Impending surgery	Hospitalisation	Wife has had hospital treatment – cataracts
Fear of ability to cope with surgery		Unfamiliar environment	
Expressing feelings of powerlessness, e.g. 'Why me?', 'There's no choice', 'Never been in hospital before'		Impending stoma formation	
		Recent diagnosis	
		Florence unable to visit John daily	
Expressing feelings of how wife will cope during his hospital stay		Does not drive – not on public transport route	

continued on page 108

107

Table 6.1 continued

Behaviour	Focal	Contextual	Residual
Diagnosis			
Anxiety related to:			
• Admission • Upcoming surgery • Concern for Florence			

Table 6.2 *Second-level assessment – John Goodman (Part 2)*

Behaviour	Focal	Contextual	Residual
Feelings of concern and worry about alteration in body image shown by:	(1) Impending stoma formation (2) Incomplete grieving	Recent diagnosis 5 weeks Insufficient/ misguided knowledge of stoma/stoma care Loss of health status Close relationship with wife Hospital admission Difficulty in fine movements	80 years old
• Disgust at prospect of stoma • Apathetic approach • Statements such as 'Why me?', 'There's no choice', 'I have always been a fit man' • Expressing concern for outcome of surgery • Concern over ability to cope with stoma • Feelings of concern due to odour			
Diagnosis			
Disturbance in body image related to stoma formation			

108

Table 6.3 *Second-level assessment – John Goodman (Part 3)*

Behaviour	Focal	Contextual	Residual
Expresses concern of being a burden	Impending stoma formation	Close relationships with Florence	Previous losses and how John has coped with them
Fears having to be a supported person	Loss of health status	Dominant role in partnership	
Feeling of anxiety and concern of how wife will cope during hospital stay and convalescence		Good support from neighbours Little support from family	
Fears change in status in partnership		Feelings of powerlessness – values independence	
Sighting, little eye contact Wants to get back home		Lives with wife. Both elderly Florence cannot physically care for John	
Diagnosis		Own bungalow	
Potential ineffective recovery and convalescence related to:		C/E	
(a) disturbed body image (b) incomplete grieving (c) loss of esteem			

Table 6.4 *Second-level assessment – John Goodman (Part 4)*

Behaviour	Focal	Contextual	Residual
Oxygenation and circulation Potential alteration, related to surgery	Surgery and anaesthetics Stoma formation	80 years old. Pain. Inadequate knowledge base	
Fluids and electrolytes Potential imbalance	Surgery Anaesthesia Period of nil by mouth	80 years old Wound drainage post-op IV fluid replacement Risk of haemorrhage	
Alteration in nutritional status	Surgery Nil by mouth	80 years old Good nutritional status at present	No experience of management concerning diet related to colostomy
Potential disruption in activity and rest	Surgery Sensory overload (pain)	Unfamiliar environment Alteration in body image	80 years old
Potential for infection	Surgical incision Catheterisation Chest infection	80 years old Hospitalisation Colostomy formation	

Nursing diagnosis (problem identification)

The nursing process is simply a problem-solving process involving a cycle of stages consisting of assessment, planning, implementation and evaluation. The nursing diagnosis, or problem identification, can be seen as finalising the assessment stage by making statements that accurately identify John's actual or potential problems or summarise the situation amenable to nursing interventions.

Staff Nurse James, when identifying the needs and problems of John, clustered the behaviours identified in assessment level 1 and then went on to identify those focal, contextual and residual factors that were affecting John (see Tables 6.1 to 6.4).

Problems identified

Nursing diagnosis

1. Anxiety related to:
   (a) admission;
   (b) upcoming surgery;
   (c) Florence while he is in hospital.
2. Disturbance in body image related to colostomy formation.
3. Potential ineffective recovery and convalescence related to:
   (a) disturbed body image;
   (b) incomplete grieving;
   (c) loss of esteem;
   (d) concern for successful convalescence and discharge.
4. Potential alteration in oxygenation related to impending surgery and anaesthesia.
5. Potential alteration in electrolytes and fluid balance related to surgery and period of nil by mouth.
6. Decreased nutritional intake due to impending abdominal surgery and pain.
7. Alteration in activity and rest due to surgery and pain.
8. Potential for infection related to:
   (a) surgical incision;
   (b) catheterisation.

As can be seen from the problems identified, many needed to be addressed immediately. Indeed, the process had already started, for example, aiming to reduce anxiety, as mentioned earlier. Others were to prepare John for surgery both physically and psychologically, i.e. the need for bowel preparation, information giving etc., minimising complications both pre- and post-operatively. Finally, there were those involved in supporting and directing John towards independence and discharge through his psychological and physical need to adapt to his colostomy formation.

Deciding the order of concerns was the next step. This process takes into account many factors. These include those that cause a threat to survival of the individual, those that affect growth of the individual, the time and the resources available.

Judging priorities is helped by the use of theories, such as Maslow's (1986) Hierarchy of Needs. This identifies basic needs common to all, such as air and water, which lie mainly within the physiological mode. Other needs such as those that improve self-esteem and role function are attended to only after these initial basic needs have been met.

For the care of John, although the needs are numbered from 1 to 8, the priorities changed throughout the stay. For example, the initial priority was John's anxieties and concerns of hospitalisation and surgery, whereas post-surgery, the emphasis changed to maintaining perfusion, fluid balance, comfort etc.

With surgery involving general anaesthetic and especially the major surgery John is about to undergo, the main needs and problems were easily recognised by Staff Nurse James, as many of these are common for all 'surgical' patients.

An obvious factor that Staff Nurse James noticed and considered important was John's age. Considering this with regard to the potential risk from surgery, his physical mode would need to be dealt with and closely monitored throughout the pre-operational and post-operational periods.

Problem 1

Anxiety related to:
(a) admission;
(b) upcoming surgery;
(c) Florence while he is in hospital.

Desired outcome

For John to show reduced anxiety levels as indicated by his verbalising and his relaxed body language.

Four objectives to be achieved to meet the above were stated:

1. to promote John's feelings of control over events by enhancing familiarisation and knowledge;
2. for John to understand events prior to surgery;
3. for John to understand anticipated events post-surgery;
4. to ensure safe and thorough pre-operative preparation.

Anxiety can be seen as a stress response to a threat, real or imaginary. It can be a very powerful emotion which is extremely individualistic. Not all anxiety is maladaptive and indeed as long as positive constructive actions can be taken by the person, it can be a very motivating force. It is often difficult, because of the complex and personal nature of anxiety, to pin-point the exact causes provoking this reaction. In fact it is often presumed by nurses that people in hospital have automatically a problem related to anxiety, where they may well be in full control and adapting positively to the situation.

112

However, Rambo (1984) states 'unresolved anxiety stimulates more anxiety' and suggests a method to achieve adaptation towards resolving this state, referred to as 'insight therapy'. This uses three steps. The first was to assist John to recognise his anxiety. As Staff Nurse James could see that John was anxious (from his body language, tone of voice etc.), the statement was made to John that 'I can see that you are anxious, would you like to tell me what is bothering you'. This set the scene in exploring John's feelings as to the cause of the anxieties.

The second step was to help John gain insight, by exploring his perceptions of the threat. Roy's first- and second-level assessments focused on why John was anxious, thus explaining the process. Finally the expected third stage of John coping with the anxiety/threat in a constructive way could be considered.

Staff Nurse James directed attention towards the stimuli causing anxiety. John did not know the details of surgery or the events that would take place, and he also indicated some misinformation in his perceptions gained from previous experience, i.e. odour from past contact with ostomists. It was important that information was given, in terms he understood, and this was reinforced by other members of the nursing team as well as by the surgical team.

This information sometimes had to be repeated and clarified as obvious misunderstandings became apparent. John, after some initial reluctance, seemed to want to talk and understand fully what was going on.

Some factors, such as the physical ward environment and the fact of surgery, are stimuli that are difficult to change. However, the perception of such stimuli can be altered.

Staff Nurse James wanted to promote John's feeling of control over his situation by preparing and familiarising him in advance with expected events. Wilson-Barnett (1980) suggests preparation is really a process of sharing nursing and medical knowledge, so that coping strategies are more effective. Forewarned is forearmed. Giving John a sense of control both physically and psychologically should increase his adaptive responses.

This subject has been widely investigated, especially in relation to pain. Sofaer (1985) found an overwhelming majority of post-surgical patients felt the benefit from pre-operative pain relief discussion. Indeed, Egbert *et al.* (1964), Johnson (1973), Hayward (1975) and Boore (1978) all suggest that nursing time spent preparing surgical patients with skilled communication reduces pain and anxiety post-operatively and furthermore reduces the nurses' work-load.

Other such information as requested by John was when he would be walking about again, when he would be able to drink and the length of his expected stay in hospital. Obviously, no exact answers could be given, but a positive indication of the approximate time span with the reasons why were discussed. For instance, with his eating and drinking, it was suggested it would be a few days post-operatively and only when his bowel sounds returned that he would be able to take fluids. When he was able to drink freely, diet would be allowed.

Emphasis on communication is a central component of nursing care for this aspect. Information alone is not sufficient to reduce stress (Scott and Clur, 1984), but a full meaningful interchange between John and Staff Nurse James would enhance this. Allowing John to participate actively in his own care, explaining and discussing his care planning, further helped his feeling of control. In fact he seemed surprised at his own involvement and even suggested that he was the sick one and should be told what to do by the nurses. John's initial surprise, with explanation from Staff Nurse James, was easily overcome and indeed as Bower (1982) asserts, John's active participation in his own care planning would support and contribute to effective problem-solving.

Staff Nurse James included safe and thorough pre-operative preparation under the problem of anxiety following the expression of John's own fears. These activities are sometimes called routine pre-operative care and address mainly the functional safety aspects such as ensuring correct identity, skin preparation, a nil by mouth period prior to surgery, consent form signed, all necessary notes and examination results collected etc.

John was also worried about Florence and said so on a number of occasions. The nursing intervention was to allow John and Florence to overcome this temporary separation and disruption of interdependence between them by allowing them to use their own coping mechanisms, with support from the nursing staff. This meant trying to maintain good access for communication between all parties. Just by talking about this situation seemed to ease John's anxiety. Because there was no direct public transport, Florence would not be able to visit daily, but their neighbours would be able to drive her in every other day. This, as it turned out, proved to be a satisfactory arrangement for both John and Florence.

Problem 2

Disturbance in body image related to stoma formation.

Aim

For John to show adaptive behaviours towards stoma formation as demonstrated by his physical and psychological coming-to-terms with stoma management before discharge.

Objectives

John to receive pre-operative counselling to ensure that he understands:

1. the nature of the operation;
2. the full consequences of stoma formation by his discharge date and to be able to maintain own stoma management.

Body image can be expressed as the conscious and unconscious attitudes that an individual has towards his body. That is, how a person feels about himself is basically related to how he feels and thinks about his body.

Self-esteem, self-image and self-concept are all closely related and if people are happy with the physical aspects of themselves, they are more likely to experience positive feelings of self-esteem or worth. In contrast, people who are unhappy with their physical appearance could have negative feelings regarding themselves (Burnard and Morrison, 1990).

John had had a relatively short period of time since the realisation of his condition, and an even shorter time since being told of his diagnosis and necessary treatment. However, he would still have, prior to admission, gone through much reflection concerning his beliefs and feeling about himself – as to what he was and what he would be with respect to body image, e.g. what effect the cancer would have on him, what the operation will mean, etc. The way John felt about his body had obviously taken on new meanings for him, and in addition he was preparing himself to experience permanent visible altered body image.

It was quite clear from his summary in the self-concept mode as well as his behaviour patterns, that his decision for surgery was based on bargaining, for instance 'better a bag and a few more years with her (Florence)'. Indeed, Delvin (1985) refers to ostomists as 'people who have traded death for disablement'. The fact that a diagnosis of cancer had been made already must have challenged John's perception of his body image.

Breckman (1981) emphasises the importance of counselling pre- and post-operatively to aid the coming-to-terms with disruption in body image. This is distinguished from teaching or information giving as a purposeful conversation in which the patient can express thoughts and fears. Staff Nurse James took on the role of listener, that is actively listening, showing John that both the factual and emotional content of what he communicated, both verbal and non-verbal, was being heard. Staff Nurse James was able, with John, to then explore his feeling of altered body image. John's needs here, as perceived by Staff Nurse James, were three-fold. In addition to his fundamental needs, he required information regarding the stoma and stoma care, he needed to be able to tackle the practical aspects of stoma management, and finally he needed emotional support, particularly during this initial stage of stoma formation (Watson, 1983).

Watson (1983) states 'A fundamental rehabilitation principle is the patient family unit. Whatever applies to the patient also applies to the family'. This implies that in everything that concerns John relating to rehabilitation, the family should be involved. As mentioned, John and Florence were a close couple, and not to involve both of them would have been difficult, and indeed undesirable.

In addition, altered body image affects not only the patient, but his or her partner, family and friends as well. Thus, the involvement of significant other, in John's case, Florence, is as vital to successful rehabilitation as are the specialist skills of the nurse and colleagues in other caring professions (Salter, 1988). As mentioned, Florence also participated in discussions. Here, the discussion with John about his perceptions to change and what the stoma meant for him opened up areas where positive factors could be investigated and promoted. Areas such as his fears of the smell, the lack of control over his body functions, the positioning of his stoma, were all addressed. John was given the opportunity to practise with a dummy appliance pre-operatively, and he seemed surprised at the tidiness of these. The stoma therapist was involved in discussions. Elderly stoma patients are influenced by an era when it was not nice to talk about body waste. These areas needed to be gently deliberated and careful explanations and support given.

A part of the strategy to help John get used to his stoma and stoma management is the use of a goal ladder. John would need to accept the appearance of the operation site, and he would also need to be able to touch the area, as well as accept the necessity of learning to care for it. This would need to be developed so that he would move towards independence and competence in his daily care. This goal ladder provided realistic short-term goals for John to meet. Attaining these goals gives a sense of achievement that progress is being made, and these building blocks provide steps to complete care, towards management of stoma and psychological acceptance of change in body image. Also it catered for the second of Watson's (1983) needs of the ostomy patient, i.e. technical ostomy-management skills.

Stewart (1985) suggests that patients who have received psychological preparation recover from surgery more quickly than those who have not. Ideally, as in John's case, where major disruption of body image is foreseen, the most sensible place to meet would be at the home rather than on the ward or in outpatients. Unfortunately, here, this did not happen. John's only contact before entering the hospital was with the surgical team in outpatients.

Problem 3

Potential ineffective recovery and convalescence related to:

1. disturbed body image;
2. incomplete grieving;
3. loss of esteem.

The above areas are so interrelated that Staff Nurse James could have treated them as one. However, it was felt worth the effort to differentiate between them.

The problems of dealing with sensitive areas, such as grief, loss of esteem and alteration in body image, on surgical wards are that resources might not be available to target these areas. Surgical wards are often busy places and, because of the nature of the workload, this puts pressure on staff to concentrate on the physical elements of patient care.

Grieving process

Kubler-Ross (1971) suggests that there are five stages of loss. On first learning of the loss, the person denies the seriousness of the condition. This is followed by anger at the situation and this anger is likely to be expressed towards others such as nurses and medical staff as well as towards family and friends, or God and fate. The third stage – the person bargains with life, or fate, in an attempt to escape the situation. This is followed by a stage of depression as the inevitability of the condition is realised and the loss and separation are acknowledged. Finally, there is acceptance and the opportunity to respond realistically to the situation.

John's behaviours, such as showing apathy, sighing, avoiding eye contact at times, according to Roy (1984, p 341) are signs of incomplete grieving.

Engel (1964) compares loss and mourning with a wound and its healing, where the loss is the wound and mourning is the process of healing. Grief is equated with pain caused by the wound. Using this analogy, the Staff Nurse's intervention would be to use coping mechanisms to reduce the grief. However, grief is described as a normal adaptive behaviour comprising stages that need to be completed, for successful recovery and convalescence. For John to come to terms with the loss he was experiencing, and his need to adapt to this loss, he would need to progress through the grieving process as suggested by Kubler-Ross (1971).

However, again one of the main strategies of nursing care was based upon communication: by somebody being available to listen to John's feelings, to support him, and explain that such feelings are natural and that it is to be expected he would feel these emotions of sorrow, guilt, anger and helplessness. John's perceptions of the impact of surgery were further explored, and additional explanations given.

This was obviously an on-going situation that would need to be approached throughout John's stay, and would be partly resolved with his coming-to-terms with his stoma. As he made progress through his goal ladder towards independence, the fear that he would be a burden gradually diminished. He was able to socialise with other patients, for example, by having his meal in the day room – although considerable support was needed here initially. He began to communicate more freely about his stoma, both to nursing staff and other patients. Generally his body image seemed to take on a new acceptable focus.

Maslow (1954) postulates that all people have a need to esteem or value themselves. People need to place high positive values on the concept of the self they hold. A person with low esteem might therefore have difficulty in adapting, especially when one has suffered the loss of body parts or functions. The question of value must then be deliberated.

This diagnosis was derived from such behaviours as John's 'concern at being a burden', 'I have always been a fit man', 'the fear of being the supported one'. These suggest a loss of esteem.

The diagnosis of cancer with a radical surgical intervention can be expected to constitute a sizeable assault on self-concept resulting in feelings of low esteem (Watson, 1983). Early studies of the psychological responses of cancer/ostomy patients reported that colostomy patients experienced fears of rejection, shame and disfigurement, leading to low esteem and difficulty forming new relationships (Watson, 1983).

The reasoning being the expected behaviour outcome for this lowered self-esteem, his return to self-care, taken from John's fears of being a burden, would thus be cancelled and he would then regain his feeling of self-esteem. From this it was important to investigate and identify with John his meaning of being a 'burden'. This process in itself directed his care, for John was able then to consider the importance of coming to terms with his body image and technical management of stoma, which proved a positive motivation.

According to Meisenhelder (1985), the perceived respect, love and approval of people close to us have a considerable effect on our self-esteem. She suggests three groups of people who can raise the patient's self-esteem. These are other patients in a similar situation, family and friends and, finally, nursing and other medical staff. However, comparing oneself to another individual is not always adaptive (Brickman and Bulman, 1977) and so the first method should be carefully selected. In this case, there were unfortunately no suitable ostomist or other patients in a similar situation. Florence was extremely supportive and showed immense sensitivity and caring for John. Staff Nurse James considered this extremely important for both of them, and endeavoured to support and encourage this.

Porritt (1984) suggests that the nurse can raise the patient's self-esteem by communicating a sense of worth and value for the patient, showing that he is truly valued as a human-being. This can be achieved through the use of skills of touch, reflective listening and an approach called unconditional positive regard, through which the nurse can help the patient explore his feelings and fears without judgement.

Towards enhancing self-esteem, Staff Nurse James followed the principles as suggested by Porritt (1984) and Burnard and Morrison (1990). She tried to communicate a sense of worth and value to John, so promoting the sense of liking him, since people who sense they are likable tend to view themselves more positively – letting John get to know her, allowing a sense of familiarity and showing sensitivity, particularly to John's hygiene needs regarding his stoma and ensuring a constant appraisal of John's needs at each encounter.

Discharge

The hospital stay is an important phase of illness for patients, but it is a relatively small part of the recovery process in terms of time spent, pain, distress and disability involved (Wilson-Barnett, 1983).

While in hospital, the ostomist is sheltered from his normal environment. Therefore, careful discharge handling is important for successful recovery and convalescing. On reviewing the research literature, Booth and Davies (1991) stated that support was lacking following discharge from hospital. This aspect of care is now regarded as a high priority by health care professionals. To reduce any possible complications or disruptions surrounding this process of discharge home, Staff Nurse James felt it important to consider John's discharge planning early on his care.

There seem to be many factors that might affect effective discharge or transfer from hospital to home. For example, one of the social expectations of the sick role is that the individual is relieved of duties and obligations (Parsons, 1964). Also, as in John's case, ageing results in reduced ability to adapt to physical stress, a long convalescence may be expected (Kane *et al.*, 1984) and this possibility had to be considered.

Mitchell (1980) found serious lack of information given to families on stoma care. Some did not receive a home visit from a District Nurse or stoma therapist. Throughout John's care. Staff Nurse James clearly placed the emphasis on communication. The clinical nurse specialist (stoma nurse) offered John a continuity of care, both at home and in hospital, as well as acting as a liaison and resource person within the multi-disciplinary team (Salter, 1988, p 193), and was a vital link for John and Florence's support.

As the overall aim of the care plan was for 'John to achieve successful recovery and convalescence', the areas of body image, incomplete grieving, loss of esteem and concern for successful convalescence, were all grouped under Problem 3.

Conclusion

Throughout the care of John, Staff Nurse James tried to emphasise the philosophy and practice of Roy's Adaptation Model. The interventions were based on the nursing assessment, and options were provided to John in formulating his care. In order to promote adaptation, an attempt was made to manipulate the influencing stimuli to aid John's ability to cope positively.

On the whole, goals were met, such as his ability for self-care, and the management of stoma, although it was felt that his incomplete grieving was not resolved. This was to be further evaluated by the stoma nurse and the district nurse. John was an elderly man, and with regard to this factor, his recovery and coping were generally successful. However, his long-term adaptation at home with his elderly wife would still be a subject of concern for the nursing staff.

In using this model, as mentioned, communication skills were of vital importance and methods are emphasised in this area. The modes concerning the psycho-social aspects were extremely interlinked, and consequently the care planned overlapped in many areas. This might be considered in two ways: as a disadvantage in repeating care, or causing confusion to care givers. Conversely, this overlapping allows flexibility, giving a different emphasis to similar problems, and perhaps allowing a more holistic approach to care.

Activities

1. The care discussed in the text tended to concentrate on the care surrounding the psychological aspects of Roy's Model. Using the assessment information taken from the physiological mode, write a care plan that would direct John's care pre- and post-operatively.
   Suggestions:

   (a) Consider what regulation/cognition systems are being utilised.
   (b) Remember the goal of nursing is to aid adaptation by helping the person to respond to the stressor. This should be reflected in your nursing process.

2. There are many post-operative complications associated with surgery, especially of the type discussed in this chapter.

   (a) Make a list of the common complications.
   (b) For each complication identified, list the possible stressors involved.
   (c) Write a care plan to direct care for each of these complications giving the problem identified: (i) goal, (ii) implementation of care.

APPLYING THE ADAPTATION MODEL FOLLOWING AN EMERGENCY ADMISSION

Introduction

This care study considers the use of Roy's Model in relation to a man who has suffered a myocardial infarction and is consequently admitted to a cardiac care unit. It highlights the fact that patients' problems can sometimes be identified through the nature of their presentation. However, for nursing care to be responsive and effective in assisting individuals, a comprehensive assessment needs to be undertaken. The use of Roy's Model to help guide nurses in identifying the factors linked with the problem, thus assisting them in making decisions concerning patients, is emphasised. The format of the study uses the problems identified as headings which enable the assessment, planning, implementation and evaluations to be discussed. These are generally put on a priority and chronological basis. However, in practice many will overlap and priorities will change over time. In addition, every aspect of care cannot be described in detail, but an attempt has been made to give an overview of the main points.

Brief background

Philip is a 57 year old man, and has been married to Susan for 27 years. They have two children, daughters, both of them married. He was born in London and was the youngest of four children. Both his parents have passed away, but not from cardiac related illness. He enjoys his busy but stressful occupation as an accountant, for a local company, which occupies most of his time.

Philip used to smoke 50 cigarettes a day but gave up 6 years ago. This only lasted for a short period and he now smokes 20 cigarettes a day. He readily admits that he shouldn't smoke but that he enjoys the relaxation that it offers. He has enjoyed 'good health' throughout his life and has suffered from only the usual illnesses. But one Sunday at about 12.30 pm Philip felt a sudden onset of quite severe central chest pain; there was no radiation to his arms although they felt heavy and his fingers felt numbed.

For the last fifteen years Philip frequently suffered indigestion which occurs after eating and is relieved by antacids. He therefore took some and went to bed. The pain continued for several hours. On Sunday evening Philip felt a slight recurrent twinge and this became more painful on Monday. He put off going to his GP as he thought it was another bout of stomach pains. As the pain persisted and caused him considerable discomfort, Philip visited his GP on the following Tuesday.

The doctor examined him and took an electrocardiogram. He observed that T waves were depressed in I, AVL, V_2–V_4 (Cardiac Ischiaemia in the anterior/lateral part of the heart). The GP gave him Aspirin 150mg, Celiprolol Hydrochloride 200mg and GTN Spray PRN, and the pain subsided.

But at about 2.30 am on the following morning (Wednesday) the pain came back and continued all night. In view of the considerable discomfort he experienced, Susan, his wife, decided to call the doctor for a home visit. On arrival, the GP immediately called for an ambulance and gave Philip an injection of Cyclimorph, a combination of a narcotic analgesia and anti-emetic.

Arrival and reception in A&E

Philip arrived in A&E at 9 am and was taken to the admission area of the department where he was positioned on a trolley and attached to the cardiac monitor (this showed sinus rhythm with occasional ventricular ectopics). A twelve lead ECG showed raised ST waves in V_2–V_4 and slight left axis deviation – this signified unstable angina over the past 72 hours and a lateral anterior Myocardial Infarction within the last 24 hours (this was confirmed later by ECG and blood results).

Philip was naturally very anxious on arrival and complained of a strong ache in his chest. When describing his pain he used a tightly clenched fist to emphasise its nature and how he felt the pain – gripping and tight. Diamorphine 2.5mg and Maxolon 10mg were prescribed and administered by the casualty officer. In view of Philip's history and ECG, the casualty officer referred Philip to the medical team on call. At 9.30 am Philip was seen by the Senior House Officer who explained that he thought Philip had a heart attack and arranged for admission to the Coronary Care Unit (CCU). Philip's wife was with him and she was clearly concerned and distressed at the sudden illness of her husband. Philip arrived at the CCU at 10.30 am accompanied by Susan.

Admission to CCU

Nurse Lynn, the named nurse for Philip, had received a telephone call from A&E to prepare CCU for his admission. A bed was prepared and a position next to the nurses' station was made available; this involved moving another patient whose condition had stabilised to another bed space. The main doors were opened to facilitate a smooth transition and to avoid delay for Philip's movement from A&E to CCU.

On arrival, Nurse Lynn and Nurse John greeted Philip in a friendly and welcoming fashion. Lynn instinctively looked at the cardiac monitor that accompanied Philip from A&E – sinus rhythm with the odd ventricular ectopic beat rate of approximately 90–95. He did look pale and appeared frightened.

The Porter and Nurse John prepared to lift Philip from the trolley to the bed. On being told what they were doing, Philip responded with a thin sounding yes and a nod – he sounded and looked scared. Philip was positioned on the bed and Nurse John set about taking his base line observations while Nurse Lynn received the handover from the escort nurse from A&E.

Assessment

The assessment at this stage focused upon Philip's most obvious responses to his condition, as well as taking into account the potential problems that somebody would be vulnerable to who has just suffered a myocardial infarction: his chest pain, anxiety and the potential that the damage to the heart could set off life-threatening cardiac rhythms. During the next 36–48 hours a more complete picture regarding Philip's behaviours and adaptation in the four modes would be collected at various times as it was offered or observed.

The house doctor arrived to clerk, examine and start the streptokinase infusion to Philip. While this was being done Susan was shown to the waiting room, and at this point, Jane, her daughter arrived. The diagnosis was reiterated to them over a cup of tea and the situation was frankly discussed. A realistic but optimistic attitude was needed to be conveyed – that yes Philip has had a heart attack and this means that he will need to be carefully monitored during the next few days, but an anticipated stay of 7–10 days during his recovery was expected. At present he does need close observation on the Cardiac Care Unit. They would be allowed to see Philip as soon as the doctor had finished. An information booklet was given with visiting times and telephone numbers, and a contact number was taken for the nursing records.

Problem 1

Pain and anxiety were an immediate aspect that arose from the assessment, which needed to be dealt with. Pain is a complex and personal experience and it is the nurse in the hospital situation that is frequently the key person in its management. The relief of pain is a major part of patient care and is essential for patient comfort and well-being. For Philip the anxiety and pain could have a detrimental effect on his recovery. Pain and anxiety are both associated with adrenaline release which in turn has its effect on the heart's oxygen need, thus increasing the risk of cardiac dysfunction.

The assessment of Philip's pain, his description of it and his reaction to it, his facial expressions and body posture were all important when identifying the stressor and the underlying possible cause. These would need to be addressed when helping Philip to use his strategies to cope with the pain.

Pain assessment

First level

Physiological	*Self-concept*
He had severe central chest pain in previous 24 hours and numbing of fingers. No noticeable shortness of breath. Dull ache at present – retrosternal. Does not get worse on inspiration. No nausea	Anxious Is fearful of its return
2.5mg Diamorphine – 10mg Maxolon IV was given in A&E	
Role	*Interdependence*

Second level

Focal	*Contextual*
Ischaemia/myocardial damage	Anxiety Unable to rest/sleep agitated Has suffered from 'stomach cramps' for some years

The problems were identified as:

- chest pain due to myocardial infarction;
- potential risk of chest pain recurring.

It is often unrealistic to expect to achieve a total loss of sensation. Patients often within the first 24–48 hours talk about a residual ache in the chest. Therefore Nurse Lynn set two targets for Philip's problem:

(a) for Philip to state that the pain is greatly reduced to well within tolerable limits;
(b) long term, to be pain free;

As well as the traditional strategy of the provision of drug therapy, i.e. the 2.5mg of Diamorphine already given to Philip, giving a sense of well-being, and targeting the pain, other strategies to help reduce the stressor of pain include ensuring peace and comfort, careful positioning of Philip, reassurance, telling Philip that the pain can be controlled, and that he must tell the nursing staff if it develops. Giving a positive approach, aiming to limit stressful situations, limitation of unnecessary activity and the promotion of sleep would all help. The intensity of the pain that Philip had experienced was now greatly reduced, and this in itself was a great relief for Philip. There was still the feeling of the dull retrosternal ache, but compared with what it was before this was nothing. But he didn't want it back!

Anxiety is an integral part of the pain response and vice versa. Therefore the two should not be separated into the implementation of nursing care and were not considered as such. For anxiety, see Problem 3.

For Philip this residual ache seemed to resolve over the next 24 hours. However, he did complain of indigestion and stomach pains which caused him to have an unsettled night. The doctor reviewed him and a repeat ECG was taken to rule out any Ischaemic changes – which would indicate cardiac pain. Philip's suggestion that a glass of milk sometimes helps was taken up and paracetamol 1 gram was prescribed. This had good effect. The next morning Philip was started on Ranitidine, an H_2 receptor blocker to reduce his gastric acid production, and was continued on paracetamol for his epigastric discomfort. This resolved itself during the day.

Problem 2

Acute myocardial infarction carries the risk of many maladaptations such as dysrhythmias, heart failure, cardiogenic shock, hypertension, pericarditis and cardiac arrest: all could be potentially fatal and their detection and treatment are paramount.

Here the focus of nursing is to observe Philip for cardiac behaviours and to recognise when maladaptations are taking place. These might take the form of life-threatening cardiac rhythms such as ventricular fibrillation, in which case immediate DC shocking with a defibrillator would be necessary.

Philip was prescribed an intravenous infusion of streptokinase. This is a thrombolytic agent which if given early in the event of myocardial infarction can limit size, enhance reperfusion of the myocardium and reduce short-term mortality (*Lancet*, 1987). However, it needs to be administered under close observation because of the hazards associated with this treatment, e.g. haemorrhage, perforation, low blood pressure and bradycardia arrhythmias, such as ventricular fibrillation and ventricular tachycardia. This was one reason why Philip's bed was positioned near the nurses' station.

First level

Physiological	*Self-concept*
BP $\frac{130}{80}$	Anxious
P 95	
Respiration 16 shallow	
chest pain	
Blood results	
Na 139	
Urea 78	
K 5.6	
Hb 15.8	
WCC 16.7 (above normal)	
Platelets 258	
CI 107	

Roy (1984, p 49) recognises that it is sometimes necessary to carry out a second-level assessment to identify potential threats to adaptation when the first-level assessment behaviours indicate little or no concern.

Both the focal stimuli of streptokinase therapy and the myocardial infarction with their potential complications would need careful monitoring.

Focal	*Contextual*	*Residual*
Streptokinase therapy	Pain in chest Anxiety related to pain and health	Unable to assess

127

Acute phase of	Unfamiliar with
MI	treatment
	High potassium level can cause cardiac arrhythmias.

Nurse Lynn identified Philip's problem as potential arrhythmias and cardiovascular collapse due to recent myocardial damage. This was obviously not an area identified by Philip himself, but this area needed to be managed.

The goals to be achieved were also directed by Nurse Lynn.

Aims

1. To detect and prevent any cardiovascular maladaptations that are a potential risk to Philip's well-being.
2. To ensure minimal risk and maximum benefit of prescribed streptokinase therapy.

The focus of care was to observe for and to take appropriate action on any behaviours that would be significant to Philip's recovery. While the Streptokinase 1.5 $\leftrightarrow$ 10^6 units over one hour was administered, it was important to monitor and record any signs of maladaptation. Half-hourly observations of such factors as blood pressure and pulse respirations would be needed to detect any signs of haemorrhage. Philip did have a small amount of blood in his urine, but this decreased and was resolved by the second day.

The reperfusion of the myocardium should assist in reducing Philip's chest pain, and should be recognised on his 'post infusion electrocardiogram'. In fact, there was only 'mild improvement' and he had developed some 'Q' waves, indicating damage was already apparent in his heart muscle.

The streptokinase was infused with no difficulties or reactions. Throughout his stay the potential problem of dysrhythmias did not occur.

Problem 3

Anxiety can be defined as a painful unease of mind due to an impending or anticipated threat (Roy, 1984). It is a very powerful and personal emotion that might reveal itself in a variety of guises.

Anxiety can certainly be observed in most people in the initial stage of myocardial infarction, and Philip was no exception. Once again, an assessment needed to be carried out to enable nursing care to be implemented.

Anxiety assessment

First level

Physiological	*Self-concept*
Pulse 95 beats per minute	This pain scared me
Looks agitated/restless	How will this affect me?
Voice has an apprehensive sound	Fear of dying
Keeps looking at monitor	'what's happening?'
Has had severe pain – now dull ache in chest.	

Role	*Interdependence*
58 years old	Seems not to listen to nurses at times
	Not usually dependent upon others
Change of role – patient role sick role	

Second level

Focal	*Contextual*
Damage to Myocardium	Unfamiliar surroundings
	Has never been in hospital before
	Chest pain
	He has been informed he has had a heart attack
	Is attached to cardiac monitor
	Normally smokes or drinks to relieve stress
	Considers himself to be a relatively fit man
	Unsure of his future

Philip has anxiety owing to his uncertainty about events:

- his condition
- admission to hospital

129

- fear of the return of pain
- fear of dying

Prior to admission to CCU Philip had gone through a harassing 48 hours of intermittent chest pain, and at one point he considered it was his lot. He had arrived in hospital, and this itself, as he suggested, was a reassurance and relief: 'at least I am in the right hands now'.

But not knowing what was going on and not being able to be in control of events were to Philip a threat. His understanding of 'heart attack' had the meaning of death or crippled for life. He was also exhausted at this point and his anxiety over his condition was not helping him to cope as well as he might have done.

The problem of anxiety was identified. In the acute stages of Philip's care this problem was identified by Staff Nurse Lynn and the goals set by her. As time progressed, Philip was involved with the problem statement and the goals, which allowed him further insight into the situation.

Goal

For Philip's anxiety to be reduced as shown by his more relaxed body language and Philip's adaptability to his situation.

Philip could be described as being in a state of moderate to severe anxiety, as shown by his inability to focus on what was happening: continuously asking the same questions, to which the explanations had already been given to him. He was not adapting in a positive manner to his predicament and Nurse Lynn needed to spend much time sitting with him, calmly explaining the situation: talking though his fears, giving reassurance that the pain would be dealt with and giving information as to what was expected to be his rehabilitation programme.

As would be expected, Susan was also extremely anxious at this time and needed to have support, and the aim here was to help her to support her husband during this critical period of his illness. Philip and Susan's anxieties seemed to be fuelled by each other, and he on a number of occasions suggested that Susan should go home and have a rest. As the day was now drawing on, Nurse Lynn tactfully suggested that at this point Philip's suggestion was probably a good one – to go home, freshen up and get some rest. If needed, the nurses or Philip could phone her, or she could ring at any time. After a few minutes' thought, she agreed. On her leaving, Philip began to visibly relax.

Nurse Lynn identified the problem as anxiety related to uncertainty about his condition, admission to hospital, fear of return of the pain, and fear of dying. The goal to promote adaptive behaviour and thus reduce Philip's anxiety would be achieved by a number of strategies. His belief of what a 'heart attack' meant was important – as he said, a close friend had died last year from a heart attack and his understanding was one that people did not get better.

He also kept looking at the cardiac monitor to which he was attached – he somehow felt that this machine was keeping him alive, every once in a while when the lines went fuzzy this worried him. His pain was much relieved now but it had recurred with severity a couple of times during the last few days and he was afraid it would come back. Also he was not used to being in hospital, being a patient and not being in control of events. This was an unfamiliar experience for him.

During this initial period Nurse Lynn kept in close contact, sitting beside the bed, explaining what was going on. She was maintaining an optimistic approach to his condition. He was in hospital and he had had a heart attack, but this is the best place for him to be. No he was not going to die, the pain can be controlled and the monitor was merely there for the staff to observe his heart rhythms and nothing else. Nurse Lynn demonstrated that his movement caused interference and the pattern to change on the screen. Nurse Lynn found Philip difficult to talk to – he seemed not to want to listen. Was this due to his anxiety state, or lack of a nurse–patient relationship?

Problem 4

Philip needed rest and sleep, as he was exhausted. The maximum rest possible is usual for patients in the early recovery period following a myocardial infarction. This is in order to reduce the workload of the heart and to promote the healing process.

Rest and activity

First Level

Looks agitated/restless
Dislikes being laid flat
Anxious
Dull ache – chest
Abdominal cramp
Does not usually take sedatives
Normally has 7–8 hours' sleep during each 24 hour period

Second level

Focal	Contextual
Anxiety	Unfamiliar environment
Pain – abdominal	Busy ward environment
Ache – chest	

The problem was identified as inability to sleep/rest due to anxiety and abdominal discomfort. The goal was to promote sleep and rest.

His restlessness and inability to sleep were obvious maladaptations to his condition and were extremely difficult to manage. Philip's focal stressors inhibiting his rest were identified as his anxiety and pain: his dull ache in the chest, which as he said was not his main concern now, and his abdominal pain. See Problems 1 and 3. He in fact preferred to lay at an angle of about 45° which was easily accommodated with the cardiac beds.

During the night the nursing staff helped sit him out of bed as he felt more comfortable there. It must be noted here that his breathing seemed not be affected, it was just that he felt more comfortable.

In the first 24 hours he only slept spasmodically. He was prescribed Temazepan 20mg for the night sedation on the second day, which seemed to help matters. By the third night, although Philip was not sleeping throughout the night, he was content to read for a while, have a milky drink and settle again.

Problem 5

Mobility Assessment

Physiological	Self-concept
Normally fully mobile	'Heart attack means life as a
Now bedrest	cripple'
	Sees himself as a fit person

Role	Interdependence
Hospitalised – sick role	Wants to be totally independent
	Fear of being dependent
	Does not want to rely on others

The advantages of bedrest during the early period of recovery seems natural, and is gladly taken on by most.

Indeed, during the acute stage of MI enforced bedrest is necessary. This could be prolonged if there are associated problems such as recurrent chest pain, cardiac failure or shock. For Philip the feeling

132

that he would never regain his independence was evident, and therefore it would be important that he could see progress towards his independence and feel confident in this. There are many potential maladaptations that are associated with enforced bedrest, especially for someone who is normally active, which can have detrimental effects both physically and psychologically. Such problems include thromboembolism, pressure sores, urinary retention and constipation, frustration and boredom – a list that nurses recognise as problems for all people with reduced mobility.

For Philip, an early mobilisation programme depending upon his progress and condition would be carefully implemented for positive adaptation to take place. As a guide, the CCU has a planned programme of seven steps, from total bedrest for the acute state to fully independent prior to going home.

Mobility programme

A – Total bedrest
B – Maximum assistance with activities out of bed in a chair
  for $\frac{1}{2}$hour, am and pm
C – Up out of bed for 2 hours, am and pm
D – Walk to bathroom/toilet – wheel back
E – Up and about, increasing mobility with supervision
F – Fully independent with supervision
G – Fully independent, supervised on stairs

The stages in between are a guide for both the nurses and patients on what can be reasonably expected during recovery and to give confidence in ability. This is obviously a tentative plan and can alter according to the condition and the needs of the patient. On the first and second days Philip was helped with his hygiene, but thereafter he was able to manage himself.

After the second day Philip tended to want to do too much with regard to his mobility programme. This is a difficult area because although one should not discourage activity as this could impose the feeling of 'invalidism' in patients, the nurse would obviously want to avoid eliciting a negative adaptive response such as this. But Nurse Lynn sensed that Philip was trying to prove something to himself. It needed careful but straightforward management in getting Philip to agree with Nurse Lynn on the stages of his mobility programme.

Before discharge Philip had completed the full programme without any problems.

133

Problem 6

Cannot pass urine.

Assessment

First Level

Physiological	*Self-concept*
Usually no problems with micturation	Feels embarrassed to go to toilet with others present
Normally full stream, able to start with no problems	
About 300–400 ml each voiding 3–4 times per day – depending on how much drunk	

Interdependence	
Does not like to have to be helped in these matters	
Accepts the need to be helped, but grudgingly	

Second level

Focal	*Contextual*
Unable to pass urine	Lying in bed
	Feels embarrassed
	Unfamiliar environment
	Has not used urinal before
	2.5mg morphine in A&E

The problem was identified as Philip's inability to pass urine, with the goal for him to pass urine as and when he requires. As can be seen, there are a number of reasons accounting for why Philip found difficulty in this area.

When Philip was unable to use the urinal in the bed, Nurse Lynn suggested that perhaps he might try and sit on the side, without standing. The curtains were pulled to allow as much privacy as could be afforded and Nurse Lynn waited outside. This did not work, Philip was then helped to stand. At first he was a little unsteady and needed support, but this eventually led to success. However, he still admitted to feeling embarrassed. Nurse Lynn took this opportunity to suggest that as he progressed he would be able to be wheeled to the toilet and in a few more days walk to the toilet.

Philip thereafter was able to use urinal while standing.

There was a potential problem of constipation related to his reduced bedrest. Philip did not want to defaecate during his first day – his normal habit was to go to the toilet after breakfast.

On the second day Philip did require the use of a commode. It was suggested he should try to avoid straining. Again this caused some embarrassment. Much wind was passed but no stool. However this made him feel more comfortable. It was explained that patients often have altered bowel habits after admission to hospital. Lactulose 15ml bd was prescribed to assist with his bowel motion. Because his physical recovery was uncomplicated, Nurse John wheeled him to the toilet on the third day. This offered him full privacy without too much effort being expended. A good result was expressed by Philip.

Problem 7

Temperature

First Level

During the second day Philip developed a slight pyrexia
Physiological mode
Temperature 38.2°C
Feels slightly chilly
No signs of chest infection – is a smoker
No signs of deep vein thrombosis
No signs of urinary tract infection
No signs of infection at intravenous cannula site

WCC *16.7* above normal

Focal

Myocardial infarction

The focal stimuli to this was the myocardial infarction – a low-grade fever frequently follows myocardial infarction. However it was important to exclude the possibility of other causative stimuli, for instance deep vein thrombosis and pulmonary embolism infections, such as urinary tract or chest, as this would alter nursing care.

The pyrexia itself did not seem to bother Philip much. At first he felt slightly chilly and wanted an extra blanket, as this made him feel more comfortable. His temperature was recorded 4 hourly: his pyrexia reached 38.2°C remained at this for 12 hours and then subsided back to his normal of 36.8°C.

Health promotion

Philip's rehabilitation towards recovery to an optimal level of well-being with prevention of the progression of the Ischaemic heart disease came under the heading of health promotion.

Staff Nurse Lynn when assessing Philip in this area took into account Philip's educational background, his pre-existing knowledge, any misconception about coronary heart disease, his lifestyle and habits, as well as his readiness to learn. It was important that both Philip and his family understood and accepted his illness, so that positive adaptation and active participation in this process could take place. This would involve a teaching programme so that Philip and Susan would better understand his illness and its management as well as the factors that might have caused it.

First level

Physiological	*Self-concept*
Weight 12 stone	Considered himself a fit man
Height 5'9" (173.6 cm)	
Smokes 20 cigarettes a day	
Drinks above 35 units per week	
Accountant	Likes to feel independent
Male 58	Does not seem to like to take
Married	advice
Likes to socialise	

Role	*Interdependence*

Second level

Focal	*Contextual*	*Residual*
Cardiovascular disease	Friends smoke, wife smokes but not that many 'Did give up for a little while 6 years ago' Stressful job	
Enjoys his drink (alcohol)	'Helps me to relax' Socialises Likes meals and goes to the pub.	'It does you no harm'.

136

Focal	Contextual
Overweight – about 1 stone	Enjoys his food. Likes eating out – business lunches
To meet ideal weight for height rating (Garrow, 1981; Jowett and Thompson, 1989)	'I suppose I could lose a bit of weight'
	Susan does the main cooking at home, unaware of knowledge regarding dietary needs. Little regular exercise. Busy work life. Gets home late.

As can be seen, there were many areas in Philip's life and life style that would need to be explored and discussed with him to open up areas of positive adaptation. Factors such as his smoking, alcohol intake, diet and sedentary life style would all need to be looked into.

The problem was identified under a 'group' heading.

Problem – Philip has life habits that are actually/potentially detrimental to his health, i.e. smoking, high alcohol consumption, sedentary life style; overweight.

The long-term goal was for Philip to take positive action on these aspects by:

1. stopping smoking;
2. reducing alcohol consumption;
3. taking part in regular exercise programme suited to his capability; and
4. reducing his weight by a stone.

Health education was one of the main interventions. Philip was a person who at times was rather difficult to communicate with and a person who did not like to be told what to do. He gave the impression of not wanting to take advice and obviously valued his own decision-making. He liked to feel in command, as was natural for him in his job role. Therefore Nurse Lynn's strategy was to initiate information regarding his health and his MI while allowing him time to reason and come to his own decision.

Philip communicated better as he became more familiar with the cardiac care unit and the staff.

He often talked to the patient opposite him, and in doing so indirectly asked questions about his condition.

This line of questioning seemed to work for Philip, and because the cardiac care unit was a relatively compact space, Staff Nurse Lynn was able to pick up questions from the conversation and offer general comments. This eventually lead to discussing directly the areas of life style that Philip would need to consider.

During one of these private discussions Philip admitted that he was having an affair, and he felt the MI was a sort of punishment for deceiving his wife. His marriage had seemed not to be working for some time. Susan and himself just got on each other's nerves. This came as a shock to Nurse Lynn, but because of the confidential nature it was not included in the nursing notes and care plan. This was something he was going to sort out himself when he got home.

Philip's weight

Dietary habits are hard to break. Body weight is essentially controlled by the amount, quantity and quality of food intake.

Although not obese, Philip could be classed as overweight, by perhaps up to a stone. Therefore it would be desirable for him to lose weight.

Philip described a diet rich in fats, sugars and alcohol, and he readily admitted that he never really bothered to consider his diet, he just enjoyed his food. A pamphlet entitled *A Guide to Healthy Eating* was provided. Areas such as his life style regarding low exercise, overeating in restaurants and high alcohol intake were all discussed.

The dietician spent some time with Philip discussing his diet and setting a plan for reducing his intake, plus giving information on a more healthy diet.

Philip was screened for cholesterol levels, however these were within normal limits. This was taken as a positive aspect for Philip and he agreed.

Smoking

The risk of further heart attacks declines on the cessation of smoking, and this risk is halved within five years (Doll and Peto, 1976). Other benefits include reducing the incidence of smoking-associated diseases such as bronchitis and cancer.

Although Philip found many positive factors in his smoking, he understood the connection to his coronary disease, and in fact it was he that took the initiative (like many smokers suffering myocardial infarction) to renounce smoking and vowed never to smoke again.

However, it was reiterated that, when he gets back to his normal life style there will be pressures to continue this habit, i.e. his friends who smoke, his wife smokes. Susan had however also vowed to give up to support Philip. The dangers of passive smoking were discussed, and as Philip enjoyed pub company he should bear this in mind.

He had already attempted to give up six years ago but failed. The reasons why this attempt failed were scrutinised and it seemed that his motivation was the wrong one – it came from a bet among his colleagues – but this time he was certain he would give up for good. He was convinced that smoking was not for him now.

Alcohol consumption

The link between alcohol and coronary heart disease is complex, probably because of accompanying factors associated with alcohol consumption, i.e. smoking and over-eating. However, alcohol may directly damage the myocardial, as well as being linked with liver disease. With Philip, he was overweight, he smokes and he drinks above the recommended number of units.

Philip's attitude to alcohol was that he felt it did not harm him, in fact it did him good. It also helped him to relax and improved his social life.

The advice for him was to reduce his intake to the equivalent of around 21 units per week. On toting up his intake, on appraisal of his alcohol consumption, it looked more like above 50 units per week. Areas as to where this could be reduced were reasoned through: such as not having to keep up with his friends round for round, non-alcoholic drinks to replace his normal intake, and leaving certain days of the week as alcohol free.

Philip was able to discuss all this perfectly rationally, although his statements of 'I will miss that. If I can't smoke and can't drink, what can I do?' seemed to reflect his attitude. His compliance to his habit of smoking might be his main problem when leaving hospital, and therefore to expect a total alteration of his life style might be asking too much. However, the points were discussed for Philip to think about, and an active plan of reduction of alcohol consumption to a target of below 30 units per week was agreed upon. This would be followed up later with his consultant or GP.

He mentioned during his assessment that both his smoking and drinking helped him to relax and this was obviously seen to him as a positive coping mechanism. During these discussions, other ways of relaxation were talked about.

Summary

When Philip was admitted to hospital he was experiencing a major crisis in his life. The disturbance due to his myocardial infarction was placing tremendous stress in all the four adaptive modes, where many of his presenting behaviours were all assessed and could be identified. Nurse Lynn was able to consider these behaviours in the context of the second-level assessment, identifying the areas that Philip and the nursing staff needed to address. The identification of the problem or the nursing diagnosis was then devised from this assessment process.

The goal of nursing as Roy (1984) asserts is to promote adaptation, that is, to increase the person's adaptive responses and to decrease ineffective responses thus freeing energy to be used in the promotion of health.

On reflection it would be true to say that Philip had successfully met and adapted to the majority of the stimuli confronting him during his seven day period of hospitalisation. Having said this, there were areas of concern.

Philip exhibited a 'type A' personality trait as described by Friedman and Rosenman (1959). He tended towards a hurried, tense, competitive, impatient life style; although while in hospital where the environment is controlled and because of his condition he was able to slow down. However, on returning home his natural inclinations would probably return. Indeed it was noticed that during the end of his stay some of the above traits were becoming more apparent.

This area of life style was included in his general health education programme, but it would be foolish to expect a complete change of character.

On discharge home Philip would still be in an adaptive process with respect to his convalescence, mobility programme and his health programme. One main area that was left unresolved was Philip's admission of his marital situation/problems. Nurse Lynn was unable to pursue this area fully owing to Philip not wanting to participate in discussions, but obviously this could be a major stressor in Philip's life that he would need to face.

Activity

On return home Philip was going to have to alter some of his life style activities, i.e. his smoking, drinking, lack of exercise etc.

Make a list of any habits in your life style that may be positive or negative coping mechanisms/habits to your long-term health.

Are there any listed where you cannot decide whether they are positive or negative?

For those that are negative can you identify:

1. the focal, contextual and residual stimuli affecting it;
2. a strategy planned to alter this habit successfully;
3. where you think the difficulties might lie in achieving the goal set.

REFERENCES

Surgery with stoma formation

Blackmore, C. (1988) Testicular cancer. *Nursing Standard*, 2 April, pp 30–31.

Boore, J. (1978) *Prescription for Recovery*. London: Royal College of Nursing.

Booth, J. and Davies, C. (1991) Happy to be home: a discharge planning package for elderly people. *Professional Nurse*, March, pp 330–332.

Bower, F. L. (1982) *The Process of Planning Nursing Care: Nursing Practice Models*. St Louis, Missouri: Mosby.

Breckman, B. (Ed.) (1981) *Stoma Care*. Beaconsfield, Buckinghamshire: Beaconsfield Publishers.

Brickman, P. and Bulman, P. (1977) Pleasure and pain. In Suls, J. M. and Miller, R. L. (Eds), *Social Comparison Process*. Washington DC: Hemisphere.

Burnard, J. and Morrison, L. (1990) Psychological aspects of self esteem. *Surgical Nurse*, **3/4**, 4–8.

Delvin, B. (1985) Second option. *Health and Social Service Journal*, **95** (4931), 82.

Egbert, L. D., Battit, G. E., Welch, C. E. and Bartlett, M.D. (1964) Reduction of post-operative pain by encouragement and instructions of patients. *New England Journal of Medicine*, **270**, 825–827.

Engel, G. (1964) Grief and grieving. *American Journal of Nursing*, **64**, 94–98.

Hayward, J. C. (1975) *Information: A Prescription Against Pain*. London: Royal College of Nursing.

Johnson, J. E. (1973) Effect of acute expectation about sensations on the sensory and distress components of pain. *Journal of Personality and Social Psychology*, **27**, 261–275.

Kane, R. L., Outlander, J. C. and Abrass, I. B. (1984) *Essentials of Clinical Geriatrics*. New York: McGraw-Hill.

Kubler-Ross, E. (1971) What it is like to be dying. *American Journal of Nursing*, **71**, 54–62.

Maslow, A. H. (1954) *Motivation and Personality*. New York: Harper & Row.

Maslow, A. H. (1986) *Toward a Psychology of Being*, 2nd edn. New York: Van Nostrand Reinhold.

Meisenhelder, J. (1985) Self esteem. A closer look at clinical interventions. *International Journal of Nursing Studies*, **22**(2), 127–135.

Mitchell, J. (1980) Stoma care in Scotland: a patient's view on stoma care. *Nursing Mirror*, **150**, 38–41.

Parsons, T. (1964) *The Social System*, p 436. New York: Free Press.

Porritt, I. (1984) *Communication: Choices for Nurses*. Melbourne, Australia: Churchill Livingstone.

Rambo, J. (1984) *Adaptation Nursing, Assessment and Intervention*. London: Saunders.

Roy, C. (1984) *Introduction to Nursing – An Adaptation Model*. Englewood Cliffs, New Jersey: Prentice-Hall.

Salter, M. (1988) *Altered Body Image, the Nurse's Role*. Chichester: Wiley.

Scott, L. E. and Clur, G. A. (1984) Examining the interaction effects and coping style and brief interventions in the treatment of post surgical pain. *Pain*, **20**, 279–291.

Sofaer, B. (1985) *Pain: A Handbook for Nurses*. London: Harper & Row.

Stewart, A. (1985) Physiology of wound healing. *The Professional Nurse*, December, pp 62–64.

Watson, P. G. (1983) The effects of short term post-operative counselling on cancer/ostomy patients. *Journal of Eterostoma Therapy*, R121–124.

Wilson-Barnett, J. (1980) Prevention and adaptation of stress in patients. *Nursing*, **10**, 432–436.

Wilson-Barnett, J. (Ed.) (1983) *Patient Teaching. Recent Advances in Nursing 6*. London: Churchill Livingstone.

Applying the Adaptation Model following an emergency admission

Doll, R. and Peto, R. (1976) Mortality in relation to smoking: 20 years' observations on male British doctors. *British Medical Journal*,ii, 1525–1536.

Friedman, M. and Rosenman, R. H. (1959) Association of specific overt behaviour pattern with blood and cardiovascular findings. *Journal of the American Medical Association*, **169**, 1286–1296.

Garrow, J. S. (1981) *Treat Obesity Seriously*. Edinburgh: Churchill Livingstone.

Jowett, N. and Thompson, D. (1989) *Comprehensive Coronary Care*. London: Scutari.

Lancet (1987) Thrombolytic therapy for acute myocardial infarction. *Lancet* **II**, 138–150.

Roy, C. (1984) *Introduction to Nursing – An Adaptation Model*. Englewood Cliffs, New Jersey: Prentice-Hall.

Other Useful Reading

Hyland, M. and Donaldson, M. (1989) *Psychological Care in Nursing Practice*. London: Scutari.

CHAPTER SEVEN

Evaluation
Justus Akinsanya, Greg Cox, Carol Crouch and Lucy Fletcher

The uses of theories and models in nursing have been emphasised in curriculum development for Project 2000 courses over the past five years. In debates about the inclusion of the theoretical ideas in nursing as part of the foundation programme for students undertaking the P2000 course, two questions have exercised the minds of curriculum development teams:

1. Is it important whether or not students are introduced early during their Common Foundation course to theories and models of nursing?
2. How would such knowledge at the early stage of their education and training be related to the practice given the eighteen months' gap between the Common Foundation Programme and the choice of a Branch in which students will subsequently practise?

These are important questions, not just to students undertaking the new form of education and training, but to all nurses, because an understanding of the theoretical basis for nursing as a discipline must form a vital part of the preparation for a knowledgeable practitioner. The practice of nursing depends on such an understanding, but a number of authors have suggested that this concern with the practical application of theoretical knowledge tends to limit the scope for the wider dissemination of theories of nursing. This is because, quite properly, practitioners often question the direct relevance between their daily work of caring for clients and patients and the pursuit of such in-depth theoretical proposals.

This attitude is understandable, however, because theory needs to be directly relevant to practice. It is a position endorsed by many practitioners and supported by educators. Thus McFarlane (1977) considered the implication of this requirement for relevance and argued that theories of nursing which seem to bear little or no relationship to what can be observed in practice ought to be treated with a degree of concern, if not scepticism.

Although such a direct theory–practice relationship needs to be established, and therefore its importance as a basis for the education and training of nurses, there are difficulties inherent in adopting a rigid attitude to such as requirement of direct relevance. For example, a new theory may relate to a new form of practice which has resulted from innovation in knowledge development in a variety of disciplines which contribute to the curriculum for nursing education. It could therefore be argued that a theory may not necessarily be discredited or lack practical credibility on the basis that a link with a known practice does not exist. This could be the case if, for example, such a theory provides a predictive pointer to a future form of practice.

Nevertheless, there is now substantial evidence in the literature supported by practical application, as discussed in this book, that a theory such as Roy's Adaptation Model has a clarifying effect on practice. Certainly, in the care studies discussed by Carol Crouch, Lucy Fletcher and Greg Cox in this book, theoretical ideas about adaptation, bio-psycho-social considerations and a wide range of other concepts and principles have influenced and shaped the processes of assessment, planning, implementation and evaluation of individualised nursing care.

As with all theories and models of nursing, contributors to this book have demonstrated that in the application to practice, Roy's Adaptation Model lends itself to the development of a systematic approach reflecting knowledge derived from biological, behavioural and social sciences. Indeed, contributors to this series of Nursing Models in Action have sought to address the growth in nursing knowledge and to counter the understandable but erroneous belief that theorising is a diversion which the profession cannot afford if it is to remain firmly practice-based.

The care studies presented in this book, while acknowledging the dilemma faced by practising nurses in applying the Roy's Adaptation Model, offer evidence to show that theory and practice are not mutually exclusive. An important contribution exemplified by this series is the avoidance of unnecessary mystification of theoretical concepts which confuse in the arena of practice. There is no doubt that those who find theoretical pronouncements esoteric and baffling often do so because of the gap perceived between theory and practice (Akinsanya, 1987).

The theory–practice continuum shown in Figure 7.1 suggests that application of theories to practice can redress the balance so that practitioners can relate to theory underpinning practice directly, and in ways that are relevant to nursing care plans. The examples given in this book clearly demonstrate that nursing occupies the practice end of the continuum in Figure 7.1, and therefore theoretical considerations lead to an application to the practice of nursing directly. The theory end of the continuum, though highly developed in other disciplines, remains limited in its impact on nursing. Roy's Adaptation Model, unlike others, such as Rogers' Theory of Unitary Man (1970), is not steeped in abstractions. As we have seen in this book, the concept of adaptation has clear practical implications which can be grasped and applied because it provides a sensible basis for understanding human bio-psycho-social needs.

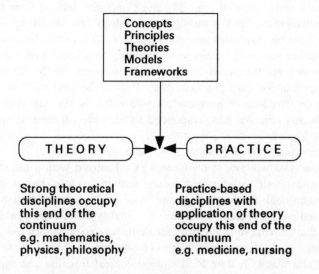

Figure 7.1 *Theory-practice continuum*

It is clear from the examples of care studies and the ways in which contributors meticulously described nursing interventions, that certain central tenets of theory development have been addressed. Thus Sister Callista Roy's Nursing Theory of Adaptation has been applied successively to:

- an informal carer with nursing problems;
- an overdose of paracetamol;
- care in the community;
- terminal illness;
- body image;
- acute illness.

In each of these studies, assumptions underlying the model outlined in Chapter 1 were tested in the arena of practice. The interaction between the individual and the environment, differences in the adaptive responses and the environmental factors influencing these were demonstrably critical in the provision of care. These assumptions underpin the systems approach to the planning of care using concepts derived from the biological, behavioural and social sciences. The resulting art and science of nursing itself provided logically consistent interrelationships between the various concepts within the model.

The application of the model, because it has many facets and covers a wide range of concepts and principles derived from three distinctive disciplines – biology, psychology and sociology – has proved to be time-consuming in practice. However, the detailed assessment serves the purpose of ensuring that individualised care which reflects the needs of clients and patients can be identified and appropriate care planned. Thus Paul, a 20-year old who had taken an overdose of paracetamol as a result of the experience of loss in his personal life, responded to the care planned using the Roy's Model.

In contrast, June, an elderly lady, suffered a myocardial infarction. She too, lost her job, that of carer to a husband with a long-term dementia. Both patients had indeed suffered a loss, however the motivation behind their behaviours was in direct contradiction and required very different strategies for quality care. Paul could see only that he was rejected and that there was no way forward. This put him in a diametrically opposed position to Julie, whose primary aim was to restore Paul's physiological function and support him in the short term. The model allowed her to do this, and with a patient who falls into the category of 'unpopular'. Julie did find the use of the model difficult, as depression is a common and unpleasant experience shared by most human-beings at some time or another. The loss of job, relationship and potential housing are spectres for all.

The depth of assessment demanded by Roy's Model caused Julie to examine her own feelings and suggests some reasons why an overdose patient is unpopular with nursing staff – empathy is easy and also unpleasant to contemplate – retreat is safer. Sadly this retreat distances and alienates nursing staff from their patients, reinforcing the poor self-esteem which led the patient to take the overdose. Paul also displayed alienation from the staff in the general hospital by stating that they could not understand his feelings, after all they had jobs and he did not. On evaluation, the model, although provocative about feelings and interactions, can be seen to have shown a successful outcome: Paul did agree to mental health care and was eventually able to return to a happier life. It can only be hypothesised that the depth required by Roy's Model allowed Julie to support Paul initially in what was to be a long-term situation.

In contrast, June suffered a myocardial infarction. Her infarction was relatively minor, and normally she would have returned home after a few days' rest and care in hospital. It was the use of Roy's Model which uncovered the enormous responsibility that she was undertaking as Tom's carer. Her own feelings of pride in a labour of love, and her total devastation when Tom visited her but failed to recognise his own wife, could be explored within the model. On a practical level the in-depth knowledge gained by Sister Saunders allowed her to make a case to the medical staff for keeping June in hospital for a longer period. As health care becomes increasingly cost driven, it is all too easy for vulnerable patients to return home to the community with unmet needs. For June to continue with the arduous task of caring for Tom she needed time to recover also from his visit, and to explore her own feelings of distress that arose. Without the framework of a model that highlights both physical and psychological aspects of care, such as Roy's, this can prove a difficult task. Within Roy's model it is hard to escape these issues, allowing nursing staff a full picture of the patients for whom they are accountable. Accountability within the framework of early discharge to the community may include making a case for retaining patients in an expensive hospital bed after their physical and medical needs have been met.

June and Paul therefore share both similarity and contrast, the loss of role function and self-esteem, and disruption within the interdependence mode. In addition to physical disruption, June displayed a positive attitude to her recovery, although needing support. Paul had to be supported and motivated sufficiently to accept the mental health care that he needed once his physical needs were met. In neither case was the application of Roy's Model particularly easy.

Sister Saunders had not used the model before and it was unfamiliar to the ward staff; for Julie it highlighted Paul's needs but caused her to examine her own feelings and the reasons for the unpopularity of overdose patients in a general medical ward. For Sister Saunders the use of the model in planning the care of John who underwent bowel surgery resulting in stoma formation and Philip who suffered a myocardial infarction presented an important lesson in how the model strands a wide range of theoretical positions. It is important, in evaluating the model in action, to note the following points in relation to the two patients:

1. In both cases Roy's Model was useful and flexible, and genuinely provided a holistic approach towards care. However, to take a truly holistic approach, as Roy emphasises, a thorough and comprehensive understanding of all the four modes was necessary. From a general nurse's perspective, much time and effort was needed to fill in the gaps of understanding mainly psycho-social modes. Although this is not a criticism of Roy, it perhaps highlights an area that many nurses need to address.

2. The concept of coping mechanisms working in two distinct ways, that is the regulator and cognitor, was not explicit in the changes, although by the very nature of the nursing interventions carried out, in an attempt to assist adaptation, these should be implicitly recognised.

3. *Second-level assessment*. In both care studies, the majority of the focal stimuli causing the adaptive need were identified, with many of the contextual stimuli that would have an influence. The distinction between the contextual and residual stimuli were sometimes less clear, and indeed were sometimes felt to be unnecessary. Whether the nurse could validate the stimuli effects or not, thus identifying it as contextual or residual seemed a little academic as these would still remain a factor for consideration until discounted.

4. The concept of the zone of adaptation (i.e. if the stimuli fall inside this zone adaptive responses occur, but if the stimuli fall outside then maladaptive responses occur) gives a general guide for nursing when attempting to identify the coping ability of the person. This is a difficult tool to take measurements from and validate in practice. Here it was left to the nurse, when identifying where the stressor lay on the person's adaptive zone. Maladaptive or adaptive responses are not always easily distinguished.

5. Roy's Model necessitates working closely with the person, in

148

partnership, towards goals based on choices and options that are available both within the health care setting, and the individual's own circumstances. This was found to be a strong motivating force in the care process.

6. Some problems that were identified were not immediately amenable to nursing intervention. One such instance could be highlighted by Philip's disclosure of his marital status, and the affair he was having. There was very little intervention that was able to be carried out, mainly because of the patient's reluctance to involve himself further, which it must be said was his right; although this could be interpreted as maladaptive behaviour.

The two care studies which described care in the community using the Roy Adaptation Model are instructive. The first illustrates the challenge of caring for a fiercely independent client determined to manage her affairs without relying too much on professional support. The concepts of role conflict, interdependence and modes are important to an understanding of the needs of the client. The need for adaptation and for the use of appropriate coping mechanisms (based on regulator and cognator concepts) contributed to the adaptive modes adopted.

On the other hand, the experiences of terminal illness and the individual's way of coping with changes are well illustrated by the second care study. The examples support Roy's view that the individual's adaptation level is a changing point which is influenced by internal resources, previous experiences and shaped by factors external to the individual's internal world. The mix of scientific and humanistic approach within the model enables the nurse to use the appropriate level of assessment drawing on the bio-psycho-social knowledge base to plan care. Thus using Roy's Model and the concept of four adaptive modes provide a professionally sound basis for the planning of individualised care. In the final analysis, theoretical ideas do not stand alone but must be interpreted and, in the case of a practice discipline such as nursing, applied in the planning of care. The model in action has proved its usefulness and its use has demonstrably discouraged routine and ritual in patient care.

Indeed, as Altschul (1979) pointed out, the use of a model can assist the individual to move confidently towards conceptual clarity and provide a concrete base for otherwise abstract ideas. The demands of the real world are essentially untidy and confusing, but the use of models helps to focus attention on the essentials and provides a logical and systematic basis for a knowledge-base approach to the assessment, planning, implementation and evaluation of care. Roy's Adaptation Model remains one of the most accessible and easily understood of the wide ranging and growing number of theories and models of nursing. It remains a major contributor to the art and science of nursing, and is a model whose applicability has been tested successfully in the arena of practice in all settings, as shown in this book.

REFERENCES

Akinsanya, J. A. (1987) The life sciences in nursing: development of a theoretical model. *Journal of Advanced Nursing*, **12**, 267–274.

Altschul, A. T. (1979) Commitment to nursing. *Journal of Advanced Nursing*, **4**(2), 123–135.

McFarlane, J. K. (1977) Developing a theory of nursing: the relation of theory to practice, education and research. *Journal of Advanced Nursing*, **2**(3), 261–270.

Rogers, M. E. (1970) *An Introduction to the Theoretical Basis of Nursing*. Philadelphia, Pennsylvania: Davis.